THE EASY PCOS DIET COOKBOOK

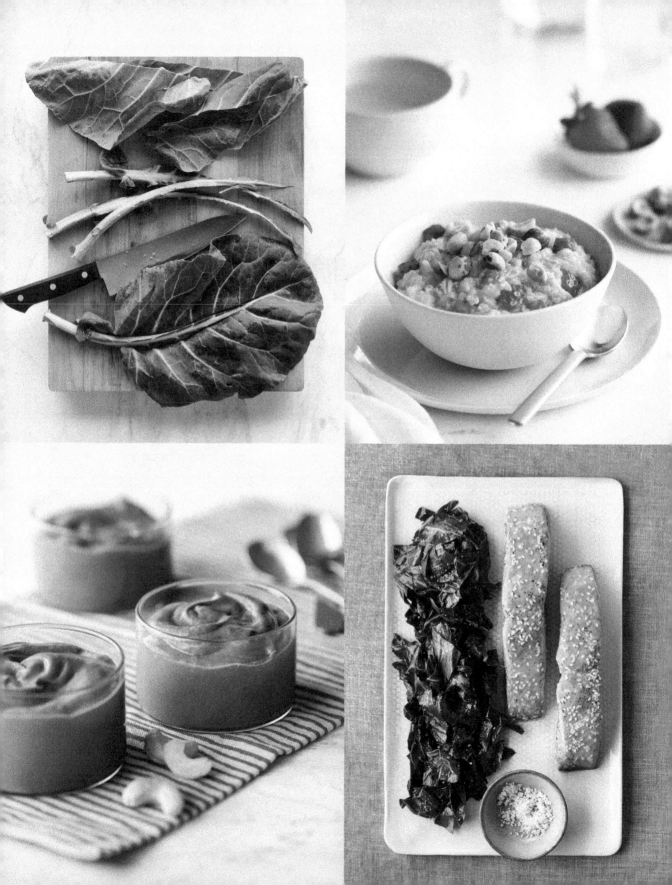

THE
EASY
PCOS Diet
Cookbook

Fuss-Free Recipes for Busy People
on the Insulin Resistance Diet

TARA SPENCER

Photography by Elysa Weitala

ROCKRIDGE
PRESS

For general information on our other products and services or to obtain technical support, please contact our Customer Care Department within the U.S. at (866) 744-2665, or outside the U.S. at (510) 253-0500.

Rockridge Press publishes its books in a variety of electronic and print formats. Some content that appears in print may not be available in electronic books, and vice versa.

Photography © Elysa Weitala, 2018; food styling by Victoria Woollard

ISBN: Print 978-1-64152-067-6 | eBook 978-1-64152-068-3

R1

CONTENTS

INTRODUCTION

Throughout my teenage years and early adult life, I was afflicted with various conditions that I simply assumed to be natural, unfortunate burdens of my existence: an irregular menstrual cycle, persistent acne, painful bloating, and a mild resistance to weight loss. After suffering for several years, I finally consulted a doctor and received a diagnosis of polycystic ovarian syndrome (PCOS).

PCOS is a common condition that affects about 10 percent of women in Western society, according to the U.S. Department of Health and Human Services. Symptoms vary from woman to woman and include male-pattern hair growth and baldness, depression, and infertility. PCOS itself can never be cured, but the symptoms can be managed. This syndrome can cause a great deal of confusion and anxiety for many women, as it did with me.

I knew that I had to exercise, but I didn't know how often, how long, or even which regimen was the best. I knew that I should eat healthfully, but that term was so broadly used I didn't know exactly what that involved.

During my years of experimentation and research about PCOS, I discovered that it can be managed by first overcoming insulin resistance through dietary and lifestyle changes. Not every woman with PCOS is insulin resistant, but about 70 percent are (Traub, 2011). The principles of a diet designed to improve insulin sensitivity can benefit the hormonal production of all women.

It has been almost a decade since I was diagnosed with PCOS. In that time, I have experimented with a variety of dietary elimination and inclusion plans, and holistic treatment methods such as meditation and mindfulness. I've educated myself on how to manage my symptoms naturally. In turn, I've nearly eliminated my acne and bloating, and restored my body's regular menstrual cycle. I also suffer from depression and notice a substantial improvement in my mood when I strictly adhere to an insulin resistance diet.

As a personal trainer and nutritionist, I've shared my newfound wisdom with hundreds of private clients. I've also authored two books related to PCOS: *The Insulin Resistance Diet for PCOS* and *The PCOS Diet for the Newly Diagnosed*. I thrive on teaching women that it's still possible to lead a life filled with vitality and happiness, despite having PCOS.

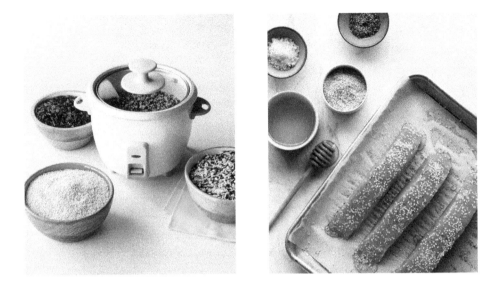

At the time of my own PCOS diagnosis, I led a very busy life. I worked 50 hours per week, exercised 6 days a week, and maintained a full social life. I didn't have the time or energy to spend hours in the kitchen each day following complicated recipes in order to improve my insulin sensitivity and ultimately my PCOS symptoms. I was accustomed to eating convenience foods and was daunted by the idea of preparing all my meals from scratch.

That said, I knew I had to make a concerted effort to improve my health in any way I could. I wish I could have come across this book back then: a treasure trove of recipes for healthy, satisfying meals with familiar flavors that are also super quick and easy to prepare.

Every recipe within this book is either a 5-ingredient, 30-minute, one-pot, one-pan, no cook, or bulk cook recipe. The ingredients are natural, wholesome, and cost effective. The book also contains handy recipe labels for those readers who are particularly focused on losing weight, fighting inflammation, or boosting fertility.

Readers who are new to healthy eating will benefit from a bonus 2-week meal plan (see Appendix A), which includes breakfast, lunch, dinner, and snacks as well as weekly shopping lists.

Every recipe within this book enables you to conquer your insulin resistance and manage your PCOS, using a natural and healthy approach.

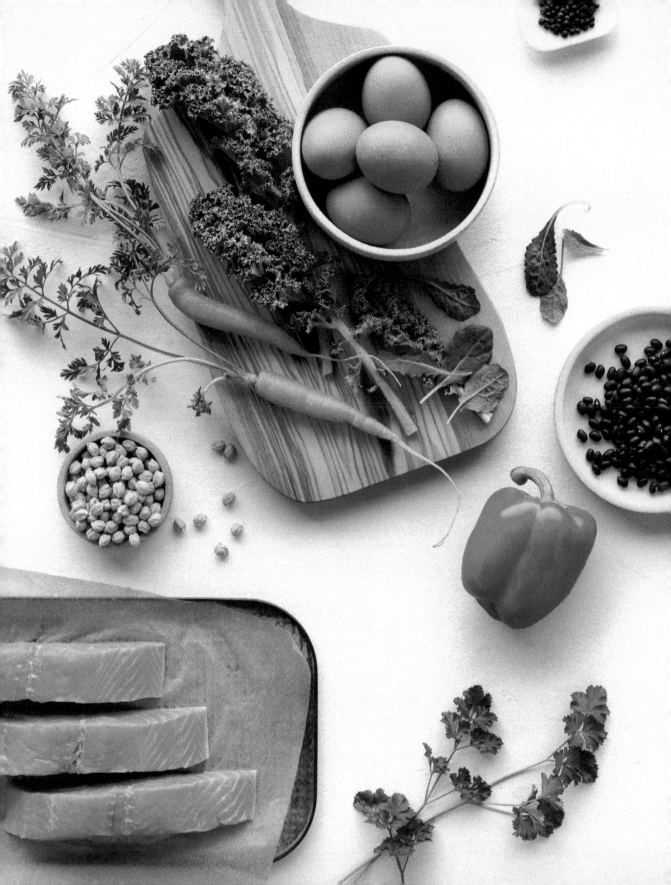

ONE

REVERSING PCOS
WITH THE INSULIN RESISTANCE DIET

Once you understand the basics of an insulin resistance diet and build some momentum, you'll see that it is convenient, delicious, and easy to follow. However, it does require some education in the beginning. This chapter explains how insulin resistance is connected to PCOS and how the types of foods we eat affect our hormones. It includes the dietary guidelines for PCOS and specifically describes which foods to eat in abundance and moderation, as well as which foods to avoid altogether. Everything you need to get started with the PCOS diet today is right here!

THE ROLE OF INSULIN RESISTANCE IN PCOS

As we established earlier, most women with PCOS are insulin resistant. This is by far the easiest symptom to tackle naturally, because it can be kept in check by following the correct diet. Making the necessary diet changes will improve your other symptoms of PCOS, so it's important to understand how insulin resistance develops, so we can learn to reverse it.

Metabolism Basics

Metabolism refers to the chemical reactions that occur within the body to sustain life. This includes the body's ability to grow new cells and to regulate the body's temperature, lung function, and circulatory system. The process converts molecules from food and drink into energy, which the body then uses and stores. Numerous factors affect our metabolic rate, which is the amount of calories your body burns each day. Factors that determine your metabolism include age, gender, weight, genetics, physical activity levels, and hormonal function (King, 2010). People with imbalanced hormone levels, such as women with PCOS, often have below-average metabolic rates (Lagana, et al., 2016).

Different types of food affect the function and efficiency of your metabolism. Digestive enzymes break down the macronutrients—protein, carbohydrates, fats— that we consume into usable sources of fuel. When we eat too much, excess energy is stored as fat. However, eating too little is also problematic, because it slows your metabolic rate as your body attempts to conserve energy.

Certain types of foods such as highly refined, processed, or "junk" food require less energy to digest than whole foods. Highly processed foods have been shown to slow down your metabolism and increase your risk of becoming insulin resistant (Palsdottir, 2017).

Eating 100 calories of French fries has a different effect on your body than eating 100 calories of quinoa. The grain like seed contains protein, fiber, and vitamins and requires more energy to digest compared with the unhealthy fats and refined carbohydrates in salty French fries. Quinoa is more satiating—which helps curb your cravings—and can produce a positive effect on the hormones responsible for weight management (Paddon-Jones, et al., 2008).

Foods supply carbohydrates in three forms: starch, sugar, and fiber. Carbohydrates yield glucose via the process of metabolism. Glucose is vital to the activities of all body tissues.

Proteins are found in every cell of the body as they build and repair tissues. Proteins contain amino acids, which give cells their structure, and work to transport and store nutrients.

Fats help form the structure of cells. They protect and insulate vital organs, regulate body temperature, help the body absorb certain vitamins, and supply energy when needed.

The correct types of proteins, carbohydrates, and fats that an insulin resistant individual should consume are explained in the Dietary Guidelines. The most proactive, nondietary step you can take to improve your metabolism is to exercise regularly, with a focus on resistance training to increase your muscle-to-fat ratio.

Insulin is the hormone primarily responsible for regulating your metabolism. Your pancreas secretes insulin at regular times throughout the day, as well as at mealtimes. This process controls the amount of glucose in your blood by allowing your cells to take in nutrients.

However, sometimes cells can't properly respond to insulin and consequently can't absorb glucose in the bloodstream. This is known as insulin resistance. It can occur when your body can't make enough insulin to meet demand or when your body builds up a resistance to insulin.

When the cells can't differentiate how much insulin they need, the result is an excess production of the hormone. This can cause stress on the pancreas because it continues to produce the hormone even though there's already enough in your bloodstream.

While the glucose will eventually be absorbed by your body's cells, you'll still have extra insulin in your blood, which causes confusion in the pancreas about when to release insulin. Over time the glucose in your bloodstream will build up, eventually turning into fat and causing weight gain.

Insulin Resistance and Hormones

PCOS is a malfunction of the female reproductive system. Women who are insulin resistant generally exhibit excessive amounts of male hormones called androgens, as well as irregular reproductive functioning. PCOS is usually characterized by at least two of the following symptoms: Ovarian cysts, an absent or irregular menstrual cycle, compromised fertility, blood sugar disorders (such as insulin resistance), and elevated androgens, namely, testosterone, dihydrotestosterone, and androstenedione.

These male hormones can cause acne, male-pattern hair loss and growth, mood disorders, sleep problems, weight gain, and resistance to weight loss.

Over time, elevated levels of androgens can also cause the development of insulin resistance, among other conditions. While it's difficult to pinpoint the exact causes of PCOS, it's often linked to insulin resistance. The latter is caused and worsened by following a poor diet, being overweight, suffering inflammation, and having high stress levels (Hardy, Czech, and Corvera, 2012).

Insulin resistance directly influences PCOS and vice versa. High levels of insulin in the blood, found among insulin resistant individuals, further increases androgen production and can aggravate underlying PCOS symptoms. Conversely, having abnormally high levels of androgens in the blood reduces the sensitivity of insulin receptors and interferes with the proper movements of glucose transporters (Corbould, 2008).

The Connection Between Food and PCOS

The link between insulin resistance and PCOS should now be clear. Aside from the medical treatments recommended by your doctor, PCOS can be managed by focusing on the reversible condition of insulin resistance through healthy dietary and physical activity habits. Unlike some drugs, these natural treatments don't carry any negative side effects. They will only help make you look and feel better.

When you eliminate toxins that interfere with normal hormonal production and increase your intake of the whole, natural foods listed on the following pages, you can help regulate your blood sugar levels and teach your body to once again release the right amount of insulin. This will improve your PCOS symptoms and increase your fertility. Learning to manage your PCOS will also reduce your risk of miscarriage, diabetes, and heart disease.

DIETARY GUIDELINES FOR PCOS

As discussed, the best way to overcome PCOS is by following a diet designed to improve insulin resistance. In the same way that a poor diet can cause and increase insulin resistance, the right diet can help lower insulin levels and reverse insulin resistance. Eating the right foods may also reduce your risk of developing any long-term health problems linked with PCOS, such as heart disease, impaired glucose tolerance, and type 2 diabetes.

A diet rich in natural, nutrient-dense foods, including lean proteins, fresh fruits and vegetables, healthy sources of good fats, and slow-digesting complex carbohydrates, is your best line of defense. The new meal regimen should encourage natural weight loss as well. It's been shown that losing just 5 to 10 percent of total bodyweight can increase insulin sensitivity (Healthy Food Guide, 2009).

When following the PCOS diet, it's important to respect certain rules to increase your chances of success. This includes the specific types of foods to eat, but also the types of foods to avoid.

Rules for Smart Eating

To greater manage your PCOS symptoms, you should adhere to the following rules.

Eat regularly, every 3 to 4 hours. Follow this rule to stabilize your blood sugar levels and regulate the proper functioning of insulin production. Eat when you are hungry and stop eating when you feel satisfied.

Avoid foods that your grandparents would not recognize. Fast foods, packaged snacks, soy products, and high fructose corn syrup contain chemicals. They can interfere with the body's typical insulin response and disrupt naturally occurring hormones. Always choose natural, whole foods over their processed, refined counterparts.

Eat lean proteins, complex carbohydrates, and healthy fats at every meal. This will slow down digestion and ensure a gradual, steady release of insulin.

Eat organic produce, wherever possible. If you choose to consume dairy, make sure it's organic. Meat, poultry, and eggs should also be organic and grass fed. Conventionally raised animal products typically contain high amounts of estrogen and antibiotics that can disrupt normal hormone production within the body.

Drink plenty of water. Aim to drink 2 to 3 liters of water each day. Avoid caffeine, soda, fruit juice, and alcohol. If you grow tired of plain water, try drinking herbal teas or waters that are naturally flavored with fruit or cucumber.

Experiment with additional supplementation. Hormonal health and fertility may be improved by taking the following supplements: Agnus castus vitex, apple cider vinegar, calcium, chromium, cinnamon, coenzyme Q_{10}, cod liver oil, diindolylmethane (DIM), evening primrose oil, fenugreek, flaxseed, gymnema, iodine, licorice root, maca, magnesium, milk thistle, N-acetyl cysteine, saw palmetto, selenium, taurine, vitamin B_6, vitamin D, and zinc.

Additional Considerations

Your daily caloric intake should be adjusted according to your goals. If you are trying to conceive, up your intake by 300 to 400 calories. This will ensure that your body is adequately fueled for proper hormonal production and, therefore, functioning at maximum fertility.

If your goal is weight loss, reduce the calories you consume by 500 or more per day. However, keep in mind that the bare minimum intake you should aim for is 1,500 calories per day. If fighting inflammation is a primary concern, focus on avoiding the restricted foods listed within this chapter. Many of the recipes in this book are specifically labeled according to goal.

Foods to Enjoy Freely

Certain types of foods can be enjoyed freely, as they do not interfere with the body's natural insulin response. These includes:

Lean sources of protein. Protein fuels the growth and repair of body tissue; it is found in fish, poultry, lean meats, eggs, and legumes. Consuming an adequate amount of protein is important to those with insulin resistance. It has a relatively neutral impact on glucose and lipid metabolism as well as a positive effect on muscle and bone mass preservation, both of which are often reduced in insulin resistant individuals (Keller, 2011).

Fresh, nonstarchy vegetables. Vegetables contain important vitamins and minerals. They are low in calories and high in fiber, which is ideal for those trying to manage their blood sugar levels. Leafy green and brightly colored vegetables are optimal choices.

Foods to Eat in Moderation

Specific types of foods can be eaten occasionally; however, because of their caloric content, insulin response, or other negative effect on the body, they should be avoided most of the time. This includes:

Low-glycemic, high-fiber carbohydrates. Found in brown rice, buckwheat, legumes, millet, and quinoa, these carbohydrates release slowly into the bloodstream. Provided they are not consumed in excessive amounts, they can help improve insulin sensitivity.

Sweet, starchy fruits. Fresh fruits also contain fiber, vitamins, and minerals, but they are higher in sugar and calories than vegetables and should be eaten with less abandon. Avoid fruit juices, and stick to whole fruits instead.

Starchy vegetables such as potatoes, corn, and peas. Eat these vegetables in moderation. They have high carbohydrate content and can put stress on the pancreas.

Healthy fats. Monounsaturated and polyunsaturated fats provide essential fatty acids, protect internal organs, regulate body temperature, and repair tissues. They are found in extra-virgin olive oil, coconut oil, flaxseed oil, oily fish, avocado, nuts, and seeds. Healthy fats are crucial to balancing hormones, managing weight, and ensuring proper fertility in women with PCOS. However, fats are a concentrated source of energy, so you must pay attention to the correct portion sizes.

Natural sweeteners. Artificial sweeteners such as aspartame and sucralose should be avoided altogether. Natural sweeteners such as raw honey, stevia, dates, maple syrup, and blackstrap molasses may be used occasionally.

Foods to Restrict or Avoid

Actively avoid foods that are fake, are processed, or contain added sugar. Depending on your particular needs, you might tolerate some of these foods (like dairy) better than other people. Also, "restrict" doesn't necessarily mean "eliminate," because some of these foods are fine in moderation. For instance, I have miso in one or two recipes. Pay particular attention to the following foods:

Refined, processed carbohydrates, including refined sugars, white flour, and rice. These products digest quickly and spike your blood sugar levels. This can cause stress to the pancreas and interfere with regular insulin production.

High fructose corn syrup and trans fats. Both groups promote insulin resistance and increase the risk of developing type 2 diabetes. The former is found in foods such as breakfast cereals, juices, and soda, while the latter is found in chips, candy, cakes, and margarine.

Dairy and gluten. Some people tolerate dairy better than others, so it's worth discussing your needs with a doctor or nutritionist. For some, these foods can cause insulin resistance and also increase inflammation, limit normal testosterone processing in the body, and impede gut health (Kresser, 2010).

Soy. As a phytoestrogen, soy mimics natural estrogen within the body. It can interfere with the natural production of estrogen and can delay ovulation (PCOS Diet Support, 2017). Women dealing with imbalanced hormones because of PCOS should avoid large quantities of soy.

FOODS TO ENJOY AND AVOID
(serving size per meal)

FOODS TO ENJOY FREELY

Lean proteins: fish (cod, halibut, herring, salmon, sardines) (4–6 ounces), lean meats (chicken, lamb, pork, turkey, lean cuts of beef) (4–6 ounces), eggs (2–3), legumes (black beans, chickpeas, lentils) (4–6 ounces)

Fresh, nonstarchy vegetables: asparagus, broccoli, Brussels sprouts, cabbage, carrot, cauliflower, green beans, kale, okra, pepper, spinach, zucchini (1–2 cups)

FOODS TO EAT IN MODERATION

Low-glycemic, high-fiber carbohydrates: amaranth, brown rice, buckwheat, millet, oats, quinoa, teff (½–1 cup, cooked)

Sweet, starchy fruits: apples, berries, cantaloupe, cherries, grapes, kiwi, peaches, pears, plums, rhubarb (½–1 cup)

Starchy vegetables: corn, parsnips, peas, potatoes, rutabagas, turnips (1 cup)

Healthy fats: oils (extra-virgin olive oil, coconut oil, flaxseed oil) (1 tablespoon), avocado (⅓–½ a fruit), and nuts and seeds (almonds, flaxseeds, macadamia nuts, pumpkin seeds, walnuts) (1–2 handfuls)

Natural sweeteners: raw honey, stevia, dates, maple syrup, blackstrap molasses (½–1 tablespoon)

Dairy alternatives: almond, coconut, and hazelnut milk and yogurt (1 cup)

FOODS TO RESTRICT OR AVOID

Refined, processed carbohydrates: refined sugars, white flour (bagels, breads, cereals, pasta, pastries), white rice

High fructose corn syrup: breakfast cereals, candy, flavored yogurt, fruit juices, ketchup, salad dressings, soda

Trans fat: cakes, candy, chips, cookies, doughnuts, fried food, margarine, pies

Artificial sweeteners: acesulfame, aspartame, saccharin, sorbitol, sucralose, xylitol

Fish containing mercury: shark, swordfish, tuna, tilefish

Dairy: butter, cheese, cream, custard, ice cream, milk

Processed oils: canola, corn, peanut, safflower, sunflower

Gluten: barley, bulgur, couscous, rye, wheat products (flour, baked goods, bread, canned soups, cereals, lunch meats, pasta, pizza, salad dressings, sauces, sausages)

Soy: bean sprouts, bread crumbs, imitation dairy food, meal replacements, meat substitutes, sauces, tempeh, tofu

Alcohol: beer, wine, spirits

SETTING UP THE KITCHEN

Cooking delicious, healthy food is much easier and more convenient if you have a kitchen that's already stocked with the right culinary tools and ingredients.

Essential Kitchen Equipment

You won't need to buy a vast amount of kitchen tools to create the recipes in this book, but some kitchen equipment can save time and make meal preparation more enjoyable and efficient. Most likely, you already have many of these items.

Must Have:

Baking dishes: Baking dishes come in an assortment of sizes, so it's best to get a few different options, including 9-by-13-inch, 9-by-9-inch, and 8-by-8-inch. Baking dishes are used for roasting, casseroles, side dishes, and stews, and of course, baking. Make sure each dish comes with a lid.

Baking sheets: Metal or silicone baking sheets with a 1-inch rim are the best choice for recipes ranging from desserts, cookies, proteins, and side dishes. Look for full-size sheets as well as half sheets if you have space to store them.

Blender or food processor: Several recipes in this book require blending or purée-ing and these two tools do similar work. A food processor offers more prep options such as chopping, grating, and shredding, but it's also more expensive.

Cutting boards: Cutting boards are crucial kitchen tools for the safe preparation of food. If you have storage space, get boards designated for different ingredients such as poultry, meats, fish, and vegetables.

High-quality kitchen knives: Knives are essential in any kitchen. Spending the money on perfectly honed, balanced blades is worth every penny. A good-quality knife saves time, makes preparation a joy, and can protect you from injuries. At minimum, select a quality chef's knife, utility knife, and paring knife.

Measuring cups and spoons: Most recipe results depend on the accurate measurement of ingredients. Make sure you have a complete set of wet and dry measuring cups, and measuring spoons ranging from $\frac{1}{8}$ teaspoon to 1 tablespoon.

Nonstick cookware: A selection of good-quality pots, pans, and skillets in different sizes and depths is very convenient. At a minimum, purchase a large skillet, three saucepans (large, medium, and small), and a large stockpot for soups and stews.

Peeler and zester: These are perfect for preparing vegetables, creating vegetable ribbons, and zesting citrus fruit.

Stainless steel bowls: Nested bowls in various sizes make prep work easy and quick. Stick to stainless steel because they don't discolor or rust.

Storage containers: Leftovers are the key to saving time in the kitchen and planning meals. Having an assortment of storage containers is crucial. Look for 1-cup, 2-cup, and 4-cup sizes, as well as a few small containers for dips or dressings.

Nice to Have

Barbecue: The recipes in this book don't require a barbecue. But some of the selections can be grilled with delicious results. This includes poultry, meats, fish, quesadillas, fruit, and vegetables.

Immersion blender: Even if you have a full-size blender or food processor, this handheld tool is convenient for puréeing soups, sauces, and smoothies with no fuss or mess.

Mandolin: If you chop a lot of vegetables this tool will save time and effort. A mandolin has several sets of blades (parallel and perpendicular) that cut produce into julienne, ribbons, and crinkle cuts. It works by sliding the ingredient down the deck to make perfect cuts of any style.

Slow cooker: This appliance is incredibly convenient. It can produce a hearty meal that is ready at the end of a long day or when you wake up in the morning.

Spiralizer:. This tool is not essential, but it certainly is fun. The mechanism creates long spiral noodles from vegetables and fruit.

Pantry Essentials

The best strategy when following a specific diet plan is to have a pantry stocked with ingredients that support the diet guidelines, and the things you like to eat. This means cleaning out the items that aren't healthy for you. You will be less likely to fall off the diet wagon if wholesome appropriate ingredients are at your fingertips. The following ingredients are common items found in the recipes in this book. When planning your meals, check off the pantry items you already have on your shopping list so you don't double up, and make a note of the basic items that are getting low.

Pantry

- Almond flour
- Applesauce (unsweetened)
- Baking powder
- Baking soda
- Brown rice
- Cocoa powder
- Coconut (unsweetened, shredded)
- Coconut aminos
- Coconut flour
- Coconut oil
- Cranberries (dried)
- Flaxseed
- Frozen berries
- Frozen vegetables (broccoli, cauliflower, carrot, peas)
- Gelatin
- Herbs, dried (bay, thyme, basil, parsley, oregano)
- Legumes, canned and sodium-free (black beans, lentils, chickpeas, navy, red kidney)
- Legumes, dried (lentils, navy)
- Maple syrup
- Millet
- Molasses
- Mustard (Dijon, grainy)
- Nut butters, natural (peanut, almond)
- Nuts (almonds, hazelnuts, pistachios, cashews, pecans)
- Oats
- Olive oil
- Olives (Kalamata, green)
- Pumpkin, canned
- Pumpkin seeds
- Quinoa
- Raw honey
- Red chili paste or hot sauce
- Sea salt
- Sesame oil
- Sesame seeds
- Spices (chili, cayenne, allspice, cinnamon, curry, mustard, cumin, coriander, paprika, nutmeg, cloves, ginger, garlic powder, onion powder)
- Sprouted bread, tortillas, and pita
- Stevia
- Stocks, sodium-free (beef, chicken, vegetable)
- Sun-dried tomatoes
- Sunflower seeds

- Tomato paste (sodium-free)

- Tomatoes (canned, sodium-free)

- Vanilla extract (pure)

- Vinegars (balsamic, apple cider vinegar)

- Wild rice

Ten Handy Perishables

These whole nutritious ingredients are common in the recipes in this book and can be used to whip up PCOS diet–friendly meals with very little effort. Choose the freshest ingredients possible.

1. Almond, cashew, or coconut milk

2. Eggs

3. Fresh fruits: lemons, limes, oranges, grapefruit, berries, avocado, pears, apples, peaches, plums, cherries, grapes, cantaloupe, kiwi

4. Fresh herbs: basil, thyme, cilantro, oregano, rosemary, dill

5. Fresh vegetables: asparagus, carrots, celery, cauliflower, broccoli, cabbage, butternut squash, parsnip, green beans, leeks, kale, fennel, broccolini, spinach, Swiss chard, cucumbers, romaine lettuce, tomatoes, mushrooms, bell peppers, onion, sweet potato, zucchini, scallion, jalapeño pepper

6. Greek yogurt, low-fat plain

7. Lean meats: beef, pork, lamb

8. Lean poultry: chicken (skinless, boneless breast or thighs, ground) and turkey (skinless, boneless breasts or thighs, ground)

9. Low-mercury seafood: salmon, haddock, tilapia, halibut, trout, cod

10. Seafood: shrimp, scallops, squid

Time- and Money-Saving Shopping Tips

Creating meals from whole, nutritious ingredients takes more time to plan and shop for than reheating a premade convenience meal. This lifestyle can also be more expensive because your shopping cart will be filled with nutritious vegetables, quality meats, fish, and poultry. It's important to find strategies that save time and money in the grocery store. Here are five tips to minimize the expense and time when shopping:

1. **Make a weekly plan and shopping list:** The key to this strategy is to stick with the list. Think about how much money you spend on impulse purchases. What about the waste of throwing expired food away because you didn't use it in a recipe? A list will eliminate extra trips to the store because you ran out of something or forgot to buy a certain item. Include doubled recipes for leftovers in your meal planning to save money and time. You can easily freeze the extra meal or enjoy it the next day.

2. **Shop seasonally and at a farmers market, or buy directly from the farm by joining a community-supported agriculture (CSA) program:** Seasonal produce is locally sourced, so you don't pay for shipping these ingredients across the country or border. Local fruits and vegetables are usually more delicious and healthier as well. Trips to a farmers market will reap wonderful results in your kitchen. CSAs are usually available through monthly or yearly plans that allow you to enjoy farm-fresh produce delivered right to your door as the ingredients come into season.

3. **Buy in bulk:** Larger quantities of foods are usually less expensive to purchase by the pound, box, or large cans. If you decide to buy in bulk, it's important to divide up the ingredients into the required amounts for recipes or meals. Package and store them safely—this may require freezing some items. Make sure you label everything carefully and rotate your foods in the freezer and pantry, so the oldest item is used first.

4. **Buy high-quality frozen vegetables and fruit:** Frozen veggies and fruit have come a long way in quality. They lose very little nutrients in the freezing process. Frozen produce is much less expensive than fresh and can be used in many recipes such as smoothies, casseroles, stews, and soups with no difference in taste or texture.

5. **Go vegetarian at least once or twice a week:** Meat, poultry, and fish can make up the bulk of your grocery bill, so try to leave them off the table on a regular basis. Vegetarian meals are delicious, and even hard-core carnivores can feel satisfied at the end of a meal. Create casseroles, paella, stir-fries, and colorful salads to meet your budget and nutritional needs.

ABOUT THE RECIPES

The recipes in the following chapters have labels right at the beginning so you can immediately choose the recipe that suits your needs. The labels are as follows:

5-Ingredient: These recipes contain five or fewer main ingredients. Salt, pepper, and olive oil don't count in this number.

30-Minute: Recipes with this label will take 30 minutes or less to prepare from start to finish.

One-Pot: These recipes are made in a single pot, skillet, or saucepan.

One-Pan: These recipes use a single baking sheet or baking dish.

No Cook: You will not have to cook any part of the recipe.

Bulk Cook: These recipes are suitable for doubling or tripling. They usually freeze well or are perfect for large gatherings of friends and family.

Fertility Boost: The ingredients in these recipes support and promote fertility and maintaining a healthy pregnancy.

Inflammation Fighter: Recipes with this label contain ingredients that fight inflammation. These whole foods ingredients are usually high in antioxidants and phytonutrients.

Weight Management: This label means the recipe is lower in calories, saturated fat, or contains ingredients that are linked to facilitating weight loss or weight maintenance goals.

Vegan/Vegetarian: These recipes will be labeled with one or both categories. Vegan recipes will not contain animal products, fish, seafood, dairy, eggs, or honey. Vegetarian only recipes will exclude animal products, fish, and seafood.

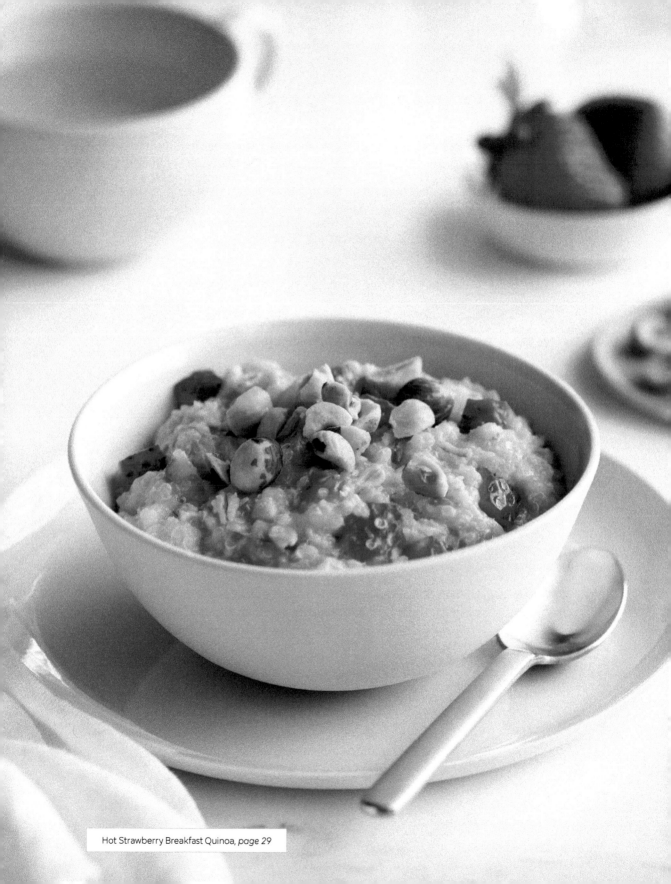

Hot Strawberry Breakfast Quinoa, *page 29*

TWO

SMOOTHIES AND BREAKFAST

GREEN CITRUS SMOOTHIE

FERTILITY BOOST • INFLAMMATION FIGHTER • WEIGHT MANAGEMENT • VEGETARIAN

30-MINUTE
ONE-POT
NO COOK

SERVES 2
Prep time: 5 minutes

1 cup unsweetened almond milk

1 cup chopped kale

1 orange, peeled

1 teaspoon orange zest

¼ cup plain low-fat Greek yogurt

Pinch ground cinnamon

3 ice cubes

It can take some practice to prepare a delicious and nutritious smoothie, so this simple combination is a good start. The orange and its zest create a lovely sweet flavor and plenty of anti-inflammatory power. Oranges contain more than 200 separate flavonoids and phytonutrients, as well as compounds such as myoinositol, which improve egg quality and balance blood sugar. The yogurt adds a creamy texture and supports fertility. It's also a good source of beneficial bacteria.

1. Place the almond milk, kale, orange, orange zest, yogurt, and cinnamon in a blender and pulse until puréed.

2. Add the ice cubes and blend until thick and smooth.

VARIATION TIP: This creamy beverage can be made vegan if you swap out the Greek yogurt for a plain coconut-based yogurt. Make sure you always check the ingredients in the coconut yogurt to ensure there is no added gelatin, animal product, or sugar.

PER SERVING Calories: 105; Total fat: 2g; Saturated fat: 0g; Carbs: 17g; Fiber: 4g; Protein: 6g; Sodium: 122mg

PEACHY KALE SMOOTHIE

INFLAMMATION FIGHTER • WEIGHT MANAGEMENT • VEGAN/VEGETARIAN

5-INGREDIENT
30-MINUTE
ONE-POT
NO COOK

SERVES 1
Prep time: 5 minutes

1 cup unsweetened almond milk

1 cup chopped kale

3 frozen peach wedges

4 whole frozen strawberries

1 tablespoon ground flaxseed

Peaches add exactly the right amount of sweetness if you want a smoothie without any added honey or stevia. The stone fruit is packed with inflammation-fighting beta-carotene and fiber, as well as vitamins A and C. Peaches also contain catechins, a family of phytonutrients that are also found in green tea. Catechins can help inhibit enzymes that cause inflammation in the body.

Place the almond milk, kale, peaches, strawberries, and flaxseed in a blender and pulse until puréed.

FERTILITY BOOST TIP: Add ½ cup of plain Greek yogurt to the smoothie to improve the function of the ovaries and increase the hormone-balancing fat in this tasty beverage.

PER SERVING Calories: 223; Total fat: 9g; Saturated fat: 1g; Carbs: 24g; Fiber: 9g; Protein: 14g; Sodium: 45mg

SUNNY CARROT-RASPBERRY SMOOTHIE

FERTILITY BOOST • INFLAMMATION FIGHTER • WEIGHT MANAGEMENT • VEGAN/VEGETARIAN

5-INGREDIENT
30-MINUTE
ONE-POT
NO COOK

SERVES 1
Prep time: 10 minutes

1 cup unsweetened almond milk

½ cup water

1 cup shredded carrot

¼ cup frozen raspberries

2 teaspoons ground flaxseed

You will be reminded of a glorious sunset when you see the color of this sweet smoothie—a rich orange with a hint of red. The carrots in this smoothie provide the vibrant color along with a spectacular amount of vitamin A, about 115 percent of the Recommended Dietary Allowance. Vitamin A is a powerful inflammation fighter, but it is also crucial for reproductive health. Vitamin A supports follicle maturation and helps produce the hormones necessary for effective implantation of a fertilized follicle in the uterus.

Place the almond milk, water, carrot, raspberries, and flaxseed in a blender and pulse until puréed.

VARIATION TIP: Any berries would be delicious in this smoothie, such as strawberries, blueberries, or blackberries. All of these choices will maintain the nutrients in this beverage. You can also try a few black cherries if you have them handy.

PER SERVING Calories: 180; Total fat: 6g; Saturated fat: 1g; Carbs: 30g; Fiber: 8g; Protein: 4g; Sodium: 221mg

PB&J SMOOTHIE

INFLAMMATION FIGHTER • WEIGHT MANAGEMENT • VEGETARIAN

5-INGREDIENT
30-MINUTE
ONE-POT
NO COOK

SERVES 1
Prep time: 5 minutes

1 cup unsweetened almond milk

½ cup sliced strawberries

2 tablespoons natural peanut butter

1 teaspoon raw honey

3 ice cubes

This traditional flavor combination tastes fabulous in a smoothie and is packed with nutrients. Natural peanut butter is extremely high in vitamins B_6 and E as well as protein, fiber, and magnesium. This combination will boost your immune system and create a feeling of fullness that helps you avoid snacking between meals. You can add up to 1 cup of strawberries if you want to boost the fruity flavor of the smoothie.

1. Place the almond milk, strawberries, peanut butter, and honey in a blender and pulse until puréed.

2. Add the ice cubes and blend until thick and smooth.

SUBSTITUTION TIP: If peanut allergies are a concern, swap out the peanut butter for a natural almond or cashew butter. Look for a single-ingredient product, and stir it well to incorporate the oil before adding the nut butter to the other ingredients.

PER SERVING Calories: 274; Total fat: 20g; Saturated fat: 3g; Carbs: 16g; Fiber: 6g; Protein: 12g; Sodium: 187mg

WALDORF SMOOTHIE

FERTILITY BOOST • INFLAMMATION FIGHTER • WEIGHT MANAGEMENT • VEGETARIAN

30-MINUTE
ONE-POT
NO COOK

SERVES 2
Prep time: 5 minutes

½ cup coconut water

1 cup spinach

1 apple, cored
and chopped

½ cup chopped celery

½ cup green grapes

¼ cup plain low-fat
Greek yogurt

1 teaspoon
pumpkin seeds

3 ice cubes

Waldorf salad is famous, but you probably haven't seen a beverage with the same name. We've replaced the mayonnaise and walnuts in the salad recipe with tart, creamy yogurt and pumpkin seeds. However, the salad's fresh and slightly sweet flavor is still achieved here with spinach, celery, grapes, and crisp apples. Apples are one of the most nutrient-packed foods that you can eat. Eating one antioxidant-packed apple per day can reduce free radicals in the body.

1. Place the coconut water, spinach, apple, celery, grapes, yogurt, and pumpkin seeds in a blender and pulse until puréed.

2. Add the ice cubes and blend until thick and smooth.

FERTILITY BOOST TIP: Although pumpkin seeds are healthy, swapping them for sunflower seeds will increase the folate, an essential pregnancy micronutrient. Sunflower seeds contain 80 micrograms folate per ¼ cup, which is about four times more than ¼ cup of pumpkin seeds.

PER SERVING Calories: 115; Total fat: 1g; Saturated fat: 0g; Carbs: 20g; Fiber: 4g; Protein: 4g; Sodium: 88mg

GINGER-BLUEBERRY SMOOTHIE

FERTILITY BOOST • INFLAMMATION FIGHTER • WEIGHT MANAGEMENT • VEGETARIAN

5-INGREDIENT
30-MINUTE
ONE-POT
NO COOK

SERVES 1
Prep time: 5 minutes

½ cup unsweetened almond milk

1 cup blueberries

1 cup chopped kale

1 tablespoon grated fresh ginger

1 teaspoon raw honey

3 ice cubes

The honey adds a hint of sweetness to the blueberries, kale, and ginger combination, but you won't be reminded of dessert when you enjoy this beverage. Whenever possible throw in wild blueberries instead of cultivated berries; they have a more intense flavor and twice the antioxidants. Wild blueberries are available year-round if you want to use frozen products. Fresh berries are available in late summer or early fall.

1. Place the almond milk, blueberries, kale, ginger, and honey in a blender and pulse until puréed.

2. Add the ice cubes and blend until thick and smooth.

INFLAMMATION-FIGHTING TIP: Add a teaspoon of flaxseed to this smoothie to boost the omega-3 fatty acids. Flaxseed is high in this essential healthy fat with close to 741 milligrams per teaspoon.

PER SERVING Calories: 178; Total fat: 1g; Saturated fat: 0g; Carbs: 23g; Fiber: 6g; Protein: 2g; Sodium: 97mg

GREEN TEA PEAR SMOOTHIE

INFLAMMATION FIGHTER • WEIGHT MANAGEMENT • VEGETARIAN

30-MINUTE
ONE-POT
NO COOK

SERVES 2
Prep time: 5 minutes

½ cup cold brewed green tea

½ cup unsweetened coconut milk

½ cup chopped Swiss chard

1 pear, cored

2 tablespoons rolled oats

1 teaspoon raw honey

¼ teaspoon ground cinnamon

3 ice cubes

If you are looking for a sweet smoothie, the earthy, herbal flavor of this one probably will not fit the bill. But you will enjoy stable blood sugar from the high fiber oats and a powerful anti-inflammatory kick from the green tea base. Green tea is packed with antioxidants called catechin polyphenols, which can lower cholesterol, reduce the risk of cardiovascular disease, and effectively fight infections.

1. Place the green tea, coconut milk, Swiss chard, pear, oats, honey, and cinnamon in a blender and pulse until puréed.

2. Add the ice cubes and blend until thick and smooth.

INFLAMMATION-FIGHTING TIP: To up the anti-inflammatory antioxidants, use a red delicious apple instead of pear. Also keep the skin on the apple. It contains five times more antioxidants than the flesh of the fruit.

PER SERVING Calories: 211; Total fat: 15g; Saturated fat: 12g; Carbs: 20g; Fiber: 5g; Protein: 3g; Sodium: 30mg

LIME-FENNEL SMOOTHIE

INFLAMMATION FIGHTER • WEIGHT MANAGEMENT • VEGETARIAN

5-INGREDIENT
30-MINUTE
ONE-POT
NO COOK

SERVES 2
Prep time: 5 minutes

Zest and juice of 2 limes

1 cup chopped fennel

½ cup unsweetened almond milk

½ avocado

2 teaspoons raw honey

3 ice cubes

Fennel has a celery-like texture and subtle licorice flavor that is heightened by fresh lime juice. Fennel is a superb source of vitamin C, potassium, folate, fiber, and vitamin B, and is a formidable anti-inflammatory capable of destroying free radicals in the body. Look for smaller bulbs that have bright green fronds and no withered or moist spots.

1. Place the lime zest, lime juice, fennel, almond milk, avocado, and honey in a blender and pulse until puréed.

2. Add the ice cubes and blend until thick and smooth.

INFLAMMATION-FIGHTING TIP: Add some whole blanched almonds to this smoothie, because whole almonds still contain the skin, or bran. The skin contains enzyme inhibitors that can cause inflammation in the body. You can use slivered almonds as well.

PER SERVING Calories: 199; Total fat: 12g; Saturated fat: 2g; Carbs: 13g; Fiber: 5g; Protein: 3g; Sodium: 71mg

KALE-PEPPER EGG BAKE

FERTILITY BOOST • INFLAMMATION FIGHTER • WEIGHT MANAGEMENT • VEGETARIAN

ONE-PAN

SERVES 4
Prep time: 10 minutes
Cook time: 30 minutes

1 tablespoon olive oil

1 sweet onion, chopped

2 teaspoons minced garlic

1 red bell pepper, chopped

½ jalapeño pepper, minced

4 cups packed, chopped kale

8 eggs

1 tablespoon chopped fresh basil

Sea salt, for seasoning

Freshly ground black pepper, for seasoning

Eggs are an excellent choice for breakfast. High in vitamins A, D, and E, as well as iron, zeaxanthin, and lutein, eggs are a complete protein. The kale, peppers, and garlic are packed with antioxidants, so these ingredients can fight inflammation and boost the immune system.

1. Preheat the oven to 375°F.

2. Heat the olive oil in a large oven-safe skillet over medium-high heat.

3. Add the onion and garlic and sauté for about 3 minutes, until softened.

4. Add the red bell pepper and jalapeño pepper and sauté for another 3 minutes.

5. Stir in the kale and sauté until wilted, about 4 minutes.

6. In a small bowl, whisk together the eggs and basil and season the eggs lightly with salt and pepper.

7. Pour the eggs into the skillet and stir to combine.

8. Place the skillet in the oven and bake until the eggs are set, about 20 minutes.

FERTILITY BOOST TIP: If you want to boost your iron intake, use spinach instead of kale in this recipe. Spinach has about 2.71 milligrams of iron in 3.5 ounces of greens, almost double the iron in kale. Iron is extremely important for menstruation and pregnancy.

PER SERVING Calories: 224; Total fat: 13g; Saturated fat: 3g; Carbs: 15g; Fiber: 4g; Protein: 15g; Sodium: 218mg

SWEET POTATO EGG CASSEROLE

FERTILITY BOOST • INFLAMMATION FIGHTER • WEIGHT MANAGEMENT • VEGETARIAN

5-INGREDIENT

SERVES 4
Prep time: 10 minutes
Cook time: 50 minutes

2 teaspoons olive oil, plus extra for greasing the casserole dish

1 onion, chopped

2 teaspoons minced garlic

2 sweet potatoes, diced into ½-inch cubes

6 eggs

Sea salt, for seasoning

Freshly ground black pepper, for seasoning

Casseroles are a favorite among busy people who want to create wholesome dishes with minimal effort. You can mix together the ingredients the night before you serve the dish. In the morning, pop the casserole in the oven right out of the refrigerator, but be sure to increase the cooking time by about 10 minutes. Eggs are an important addition to your diet if you want to reduce inflammation and boost fertility. Eggs are high in vitamin D, which can diminish inflammation and help create the hormones that support healthy ovulation.

1. Preheat the oven to 350°F.

2. Lightly oil an 8-by-8-inch baking dish and set aside.

3. Heat the olive oil in a large skillet over medium-high heat.

4. Add the onion, garlic, and sweet potatoes and sauté for 10 minutes, until the vegetables are just cooked through.

5. Spread the sweet potato mixture in the bottom of the casserole dish.

6. In a medium bowl, whisk the eggs and season them lightly with salt and pepper.

7. Pour the eggs into the casserole dish and bake until the eggs are cooked and firm, about 40 minutes.

INFLAMMATION-FIGHTING TIP: Add 1 cup shredded spinach to the eggs before pouring them into the casserole dish. Spinach is rich in carotenoids as well as vitamins C, E, and K—all of which can protect the body from inflammation.

PER SERVING Calories: 183; Total fat: 9g; Saturated fat: 2g; Carbs: 16g; Fiber: 3g; Protein: 10g; Sodium: 129mg

NAVY BEAN EGG SCRAMBLE

FERTILITY BOOST • INFLAMMATION FIGHTER • WEIGHT MANAGEMENT • VEGETARIAN

5-INGREDIENT
30-MINUTE
ONE-POT

SERVES 4
Prep time: 10 minutes
Cook time: 15 minutes

2 teaspoons olive oil

2 cups sodium-free canned navy beans, rinsed and drained

8 eggs, beaten

½ cup prepared salsa

½ avocado, diced

1 tablespoon chopped fresh cilantro

This colorful meal is basically a simple version of huevos rancheros that can be quickly put in front of family and guests. Look for sodium-free prepared salsa or make your own if you have a favorite recipe and a little extra time. The avocado adds a rich and creamy texture along with healthy fats, which are crucial for hormone production and fertility.

1. Heat the olive oil in a large skillet over medium heat.

2. Add the beans and sauté for about 5 minutes, until the beans are heated through.

3. Stir in the eggs and as they begin to set, gently pull them across the skillet with a spatula to form large soft curds. Continue cooking the eggs until no visible liquid egg remains, about 8 minutes.

4. Serve the eggs topped with salsa, avocado, and cilantro.

VARIATION TIP: Wrap the eggs, salsa, beans, avocado, and cilantro in sprouted grain tortillas for a more filling and portable meal. On a busy day you can make the wrap ahead of time and eat it while on the run.

PER SERVING Calories: 333; Total fat: 16g; Saturated fat: 4g; Carbs: 28g; Fiber: 12g; Protein: 20g; Sodium: 280mg

HOT STRAWBERRY BREAKFAST QUINOA

INFLAMMATION FIGHTER • WEIGHT MANAGEMENT • VEGAN/VEGETARIAN

5-INGREDIENT
30-MINUTE
ONE-POT

SERVES 4
Prep time: 5 minutes
Cook time: 20 minutes

2 cups water

1 cup unsweetened almond milk

1 teaspoon pure vanilla extract

½ cup quinoa

½ cup rolled oats

Pinch sea salt

1 cup sliced fresh strawberries, sliced

Start off your day with this comforting and substantial hot cereal. Quinoa combined with oatmeal adds a creamy, nutty flavor to the sweetness of the strawberries. Pure vanilla extract is not only delicious; it also contains vanillic acid and vanillin, two inflammation busting antioxidants. For a truly luscious vanilla taste, scrape the seeds from half a vanilla bean into the almond milk instead of using the extract.

1. In a medium pot, stir together the water, almond milk, vanilla, quinoa, oats, and salt over medium-high heat.

2. Bring the mixture to a boil and then reduce the heat to low and simmer for 20 minutes. Stir frequently until the grains are tender and the cereal is thick and creamy.

3. Remove the cereal from the heat and stir in the strawberries.

FERTILITY BOOST TIP: Add ¼ cup chopped hazelnuts to this hot cereal for a lovely crunch and nutrition boost. Hazelnuts are high in folic acid and healthy omega-3 fatty acids; both are crucial for preventing birth defects. Toast the hazelnuts lightly in a 250°F oven to deepen the flavor before chopping them.

PER SERVING Calories: 161; Total fat: 5g; Saturated fat: 1g; Carbs: 22g; Fiber: 4g; Protein: 5g; Sodium: 87mg

PEACH, NUT, AND SUNFLOWER SEED MUESLI

FERTILITY BOOST • WEIGHT MANAGEMENT • VEGETARIAN

ONE-POT
NO COOK
BULK COOK

SERVES 4
Prep time: 5 minutes,
plus 30 minutes of
refrigeration time

½ cup rolled oats

¼ cup sunflower seeds

¼ cup almond slivers

2 tablespoons chia seeds

2 tablespoons chopped
hazelnuts

2 tablespoons flaxseed

½ teaspoon ground
cinnamon

1 cup plain low-fat
Greek yogurt

½ cup unsweetened
almond milk

2 peaches, chopped

The specific seeds, nuts, and fruit listed here are just a suggestion. Feel free to use your favorites in similar amounts to make a satisfying breakfast. The peaches contain antioxidants such as vitamin A, vitamin C, and beta-carotene. Vitamin C can help regulate ovarian function and the menstrual cycle as well as boost hormone health. The vitamin A in this fragrant fruit can support conception by helping the follicles mature. Almonds are a good source of magnesium, which can improve insulin resistance.

1. In a medium bowl, stir together the oats, sunflower seeds, almonds, chia seeds, hazelnuts, flaxseed, and cinnamon until well mixed.

2. Stir in the yogurt and almond milk and refrigerate the muesli for at least 30 minutes, up to 1 hour.

3. Serve topped with peaches.

BULK COOKING TIP: This isn't a recipe you can freeze after adding the yogurt, milk, and fruit. But you can make a double batch easily to feed extra guests. The seed, nuts, and oatmeal mixture can be made in a large amount and stored in a sealed container in your cupboard for up to a month. Simply scoop out the desired amount of dry ingredients and add the wet ingredients as needed.

PER SERVING Calories: 234; Total fat: 11g; Saturated fat: 2g; Carbs: 24g; Fiber: 7g; Protein: 10g; Sodium: 68mg

MUSHROOM VEGGIE HASH

INFLAMMATION FIGHTER • WEIGHT MANAGEMENT • VEGETARIAN

ONE-POT

SERVES 4
Prep time: 10 minutes
Cook time: 30 minutes

1 tablespoon olive oil

1 sweet onion, chopped

2 teaspoons minced garlic

½ pound Brussels sprouts, sliced

2 cups sliced wild mushrooms

1 red bell pepper, chopped

2 teaspoons chopped fresh thyme

Sea salt, for seasoning

Freshly ground black pepper, for seasoning

4 eggs

Most of us don't have the time to forage for wild mushrooms—or likely even live in an area where these fungi grow. Luckily you can find many mushroom varieties such as oyster, chanterelles, and morels in the grocery store. Wild mushrooms are an excellent source of inflammation fighting antioxidants, including selenium, vitamin D, fiber, potassium, and vitamin C. Mushrooms are good at making you feel full, which can reduce calorie consumption and support a healthy immune system.

1. Preheat the oven to 400°F.

2. Heat the olive oil in a large oven-safe skillet over medium-high heat.

3. Add the onion and garlic and sauté for about 3 minutes, until softened.

4. Add the Brussels sprouts, mushrooms, red bell pepper, and thyme and sauté until the vegetables are lightly caramelized, about 15 minutes.

5. Season the veggies lightly with salt and pepper.

6. Make four wells in the vegetables and crack the eggs into the wells.

7. Place the skillet in the oven and bake until the eggs are cooked through, about 10 minutes.

INGREDIENT TIP: Brussels sprouts have woody, unpalatable stems, so be sure to cut them off. Trim about ½ inch off the bottom of each sprout before washing and slicing them thinly for this hash.

PER SERVING Calories: 149; Total fat: 8g; Saturated fat: 2g; Carbs: 12g; Fiber: 4g; Protein: 9g; Sodium: 139mg

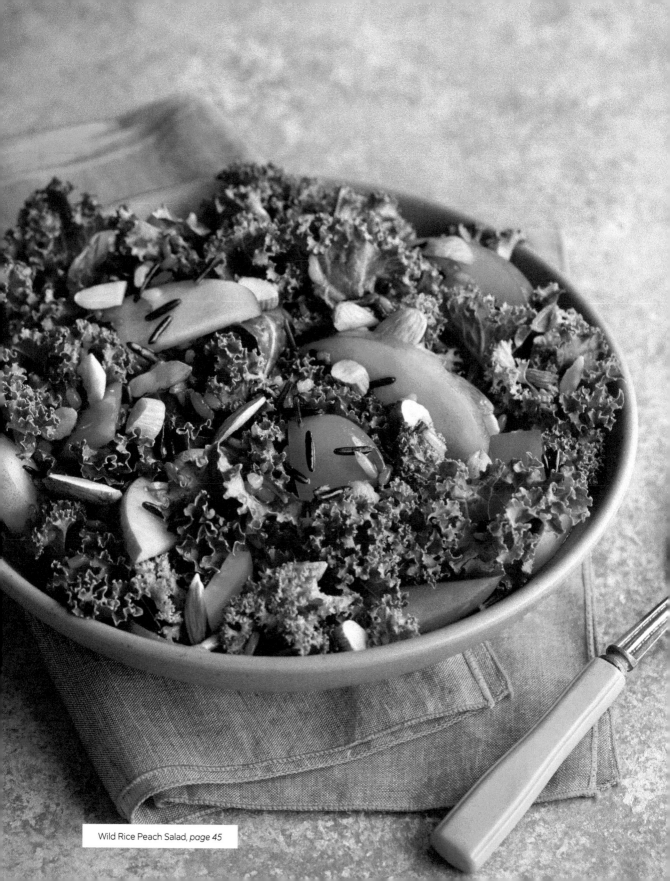

Wild Rice Peach Salad, *page 45*

SIMPLE TOMATO SOUP

INFLAMMATION FIGHTER • WEIGHT MANAGEMENT

5-INGREDIENT
30-MINUTE
BULK COOK

SERVES 4
Prep time: 10 minutes
Cook time: 20 minutes

1 tablespoon olive oil

1 small onion, chopped

1 tablespoon
minced garlic

2 (28-ounce) cans
sodium-free diced
tomatoes

4 cups sodium-free
chicken broth

1 tablespoon dried
Italian seasoning

Sea salt, for seasoning

Freshly ground black
pepper, for seasoning

Tomato soup is the basis of many happy childhood lunches, although some people have only tasted the inferior canned version. Tomatoes gain even greater health benefits when cooked, because the heat increases the availability of lycopene, a phytochemical that is a powerful antioxidant. Tomatoes are also very high in vitamins A, C, and E.

1. Heat the olive oil in a large saucepan over medium-high heat.

2. Add the onion and garlic and sauté until softened, about 3 minutes.

3. Stir in the tomatoes, broth, and Italian seasoning and bring the soup to a boil.

4. Reduce the heat to low and simmer 15 minutes.

5. Use an immersion blender to purée the soup or transfer the soup to a blender or food processor and pulse until smooth.

6. Return the soup to the saucepan and season with salt and pepper.

BULK COOKING TIP: This soup freezes beautifully. Be sure to completely cool it down in the refrigerator before freezing.

PER SERVING Calories: 146; Total fat: 16g; Saturated fat: 1g; Carbs: 15g; Fiber: 3g; Protein: 7g; Sodium: 162mg

EASY SPLIT PEA SOUP

INFLAMMATION FIGHTER • WEIGHT MANAGEMENT

5-INGREDIENT
ONE-POT
BULK COOK

SERVES 4
Prep time: 10 minutes
Cook time: 2 hours and
30 minutes

1 tablespoon olive oil

1 sweet onion, chopped

4 celery stalks, chopped

2 teaspoons minced garlic

6 cups sodium-free
chicken broth

1½ cups dried split peas,
picked through

Sea salt, for seasoning

Freshly ground black
pepper, for seasoning

Split pea soup is a comfort food that is usually consumed during cold-weather months, preferably out of a thick pottery mug while covered by a fleecy blanket. The stick-to-your-ribs texture of the soup evokes these types of images. Of course, pea soup can be enjoyed year-round and should be; it is packed with fiber that can lower your blood sugar, along with B vitamins and protein.

1. Heat the olive oil in a large saucepan over medium-high heat.

2. Add the onion, celery, and garlic and sauté until softened, about 5 minutes.

3. Add the chicken stock and peas and bring the soup to a boil.

4. Reduce the heat to low and simmer until the peas are very tender and the soup is thick, about 2 to 2½ hours.

5. Season the soup with salt and pepper.

BULK COOKING TIP: This soup holds up well when frozen, so go ahead and double the recipe. As the soup chills it will also thicken, so it is best to store it in a sealable plastic freezer bag instead of a container. Add a little extra broth when reheating, to achieve the desired texture.

PER SERVING Calories: 350; Total fat: 25g; Saturated fat: 1g; Carbs: 45g; Fiber: 21g; Protein: 26g; Sodium: 221mg

GOLDEN BUTTERNUT SQUASH SOUP

FERTILITY BOOST • INFLAMMATION FIGHTER • WEIGHT MANAGEMENT • VEGAN/VEGETARIAN

5-INGREDIENT

SERVES 4
Prep time: 10 minutes
Cook time: 35 minutes

1 tablespoon olive oil

1 sweet onion, chopped

1 medium butternut squash, peeled and diced into ½-inch chunks

6 cups sodium-free vegetable broth

1 teaspoon ground nutmeg

½ cup coconut milk

Sea salt, for seasoning

This elegant soup has a velvety smooth texture and a beautiful bright color. Squash is one of those naturally sweet vegetables that can be prepared with warm spices such as cloves or cinnamon. It is also one of the best sources of inflammation fighting antioxidants such as alpha-carotene, beta-carotene, lutein, zeaxanthin, and beta-cryptoxanthin. The starch in this vegetable is made up of polysaccharides that have anti-inflammatory properties and can help regulate insulin.

1. Heat the olive oil in a large saucepan over medium-high heat.

2. Add the onion and sauté until softened, about 3 minutes.

3. Stir in the squash, broth, and nutmeg and bring the soup to a boil.

4. Reduce the heat to low and simmer until the squash is very tender, about 30 minutes.

5. Purée the soup in a food processor or blender and return to the saucepan, or use an immersion bender.

6. Stir in the coconut milk.

7. Season with salt and serve.

INFLAMMATION-FIGHTING TIP: Add 1 tablespoon grated fresh ginger to this soup for a kick of flavor and a powerful anti-inflammatory compound called gingerol. This compound blocks enzymes and genes in the body that increase inflammation.

PER SERVING Calories: 185; Total fat: 11g; Saturated fat: 7g; Carbs: 21g; Fiber: 5g; Protein: 4g; Sodium: 457mg

HEARTY CHICKEN MINESTRONE

FERTILITY BOOST • INFLAMMATION FIGHTER • WEIGHT MANAGEMENT

ONE-POT
BULK COOK

SERVES 8
Prep time: 15 minutes
Cook time: 50 minutes

1 tablespoon olive oil

1 sweet onion, chopped

1 tablespoon
minced garlic

4 celery stalks with the
greens, chopped

2 cups shredded cabbage

1 (28-ounce) can
sodium-free diced
tomatoes

6 cups sodium-free
chicken stock

2 cups chopped
cooked chicken

4 cups spinach

1 tablespoon dried Italian
seasoning

Sea salt, for seasoning

Freshly ground black
pepper, for seasoning

The vegetables in this soup are so plentiful you might need to buy bigger bowls! Cabbage adds glutamine, an amino acid, and vitamin C, which can boost the immune system and fight inflammation. Chop up a few extra stalks of celery to increase the amount of diindolylmethane (DIM) a phytonutrient that can reduce the risk of endometriosis and fibroids.

1. Heat the olive oil in a large stockpot over medium-high heat.

2. Add the onion and garlic and sauté for about 3 minutes, until softened.

3. Stir in the celery and cabbage and sauté for 5 minutes.

4. Stir in the diced tomatoes and chicken stock and bring the soup to a boil.

5. Reduce the heat to low and simmer the soup until the vegetables are tender, about 35 minutes.

6. Stir in the chicken, spinach, and the Italian seasoning and simmer until the chicken is heated through and the spinach is wilted, about 5 minutes.

7. Season the soup with salt and pepper.

BULK COOKING TIP: If you plan to freeze portions of this comforting soup, wait to add the spinach until after you portion it out. The spinach should be stirred in when you reheat the soup so that the greens retain their color and texture.

PER SERVING Calories: 101; Total fat: 3g; Saturated fat: 1g; Carbs: 10g; Fiber: 2g; Protein: 12g; Sodium: 206mg

MULLIGATAWNY SOUP

FERTILITY BOOST • INFLAMMATION FIGHTER • WEIGHT MANAGEMENT • VEGAN/VEGETARIAN

ONE-POT
BULK COOK

SERVES 8
Prep time: 10 minutes
Cook time: 50 minutes

2 tablespoons olive oil

1 sweet onion, chopped

2 teaspoons minced garlic

2 teaspoons grated
fresh ginger

3 tablespoons
curry powder

6 cups sodium-free
vegetable stock

1½ cups red lentils, rinsed

1 (15-ounce) can
sodium-free chickpeas

Juice and zest of 1 lemon

2 cups chopped kale

Sea salt, for seasoning

Freshly ground
black pepper

Mulligatawny is loosely translated to "pepper water." The name is appropriate because this modern soup has a generous amount of spicing, about six types. This version is vegetarian, but chicken and lamb are also traditional ingredients. The lemon juice brightens the flavor of the lentils and chickpeas, creating a fresh, satisfying meal. Add a little extra cayenne if you like to turn up the heat in your recipes.

1. In a large stockpot over medium-high heat, heat the olive oil.

2. Add the onion, garlic, and ginger and sauté for about 3 minutes, until softened.

3. Stir in the curry powder and sauté for about 2 minutes until fragrant.

4. Add the vegetable stock, lentils, chickpeas, lemon juice, and zest.

5. Bring the soup to a boil and then reduce the heat to low and simmer for about 40 minutes, until the lentils are soft and the soup is thick.

6. Stir in the kale and simmer for about 4 minutes, until it's wilted

7. Season the soup with salt and pepper.

BULK COOKING TIP: The aromatic, warm spices in this traditional soup will mellow and deepen as the soup is stored in the refrigerator. If you want to freeze portions, wait until the second day so the ingredients have time to blend and create the perfect balance of flavors.

PER SERVING Calories: 141; Total fat: 5g; Saturated fat: 1g; Carbs: 19g; Fiber: 6g; Protein: 7g; Sodium: 121mg

COCONUT-GINGER SOUP

FERTILITY BOOST • INFLAMMATION FIGHTER • VEGAN/VEGETARIAN

ONE-POT
30-MINUTE

SERVES 4
Prep time: 10 minutes
Cook time: 20 minutes

1 tablespoon coconut oil

1 sweet onion, chopped

1 tablespoon grated
fresh ginger

2 teaspoons minced garlic

4 celery stalks, chopped

1 tablespoon
ground cumin

6 cups sodium-free
vegetable stock

1 (15-ounce) can
sodium-free navy beans

1 cup coconut milk

4 cups chopped kale

Sea salt, for seasoning

Freshly ground black
pepper, for seasoning

Some ingredients are used so regularly in recipes it's easy to forget they have important health benefits of their own. Celery is one of these humble, overlooked ingredients. It is an excellent source of manganese, calcium, phosphorus, beta-carotene, and vitamin C, and can reduce the damage caused by free radicals.

1. Heat the coconut oil in a large stockpot over medium-high heat.

2. Add the onion, ginger, and garlic and sauté for about 3 minutes, until softened.

3. Stir in the celery and cumin and sauté for 4 minutes.

4. Add in the vegetable stock and navy beans and bring the soup to a boil.

5. Reduce the heat to low and simmer for 10 minutes.

6. Remove the soup from the heat and use an immersion blender or blender to purée the soup smooth.

7. Return the soup to the heat and stir in the coconut milk and kale.

8. Heat for about 3 minutes, until the kale wilts.

9. Season the soup with salt and pepper and serve.

WEIGHT MANAGEMENT TIP: Cut the coconut milk by ½ cup to reduce the calories by 50, the total fat by 4 grams and saturated fat by 4 grams per serving. The soup will still be creamy and delicious.

PER SERVING Calories: 372; Total fat: 20g; Saturated fat: 16g; Carbs: 40g; Fiber: 15g; Protein: 14g; Sodium: 298mg

RED LENTIL POTTAGE

INFLAMMATION FIGHTER • WEIGHT MANAGEMENT • VEGAN/VEGETARIAN

ONE-POT
BULK COOK

SERVES 4
Prep time: 10 minutes
Cook time: 1 hour

1 tablespoon olive oil

1 sweet onion, chopped

2 celery stalks with greens, sliced

1 tablespoon minced garlic

6 cups sodium-free vegetable stock

4 cups red lentils, rinsed

2 teaspoons ground cumin

Sea salt, for seasoning

Freshly ground black pepper, for seasoning

A pottage is a thick soup kept bubbling on the stove for several days. It was a staple for peasants, centuries past, who only had access to inexpensive ingredients. Lentils are the perfect base for this meal because they are packed with nutrients such as fiber, which can stabilize blood sugar. Lentils are also very high in iron, folate, copper, molybdenum, and protein.

1. Heat the olive oil in a large stockpot over medium-high heat.

2. Add the onion, celery, and garlic and sauté for 4 to 5 minutes, until they're translucent.

3. Stir in the stock, lentils, and cumin and bring the soup to a boil.

4. Reduce the heat to low and simmer, covered, for 45 to 50 minutes, until the lentils are tender.

5. Remove the soup from the heat and season with salt and pepper.

BULK COOKING TIP: When doubling the recipe, keep the garlic and cumin at the same amounts; doubling them will only overpower the other ingredients.

PER SERVING Calories: 257; Total fat: 4g; Saturated fat: 1g; Carbs: 39g; Fiber: 19g; Protein: 16g; Sodium: 234mg

CREAM OF WATERCRESS AND KALE SOUP

INFLAMMATION FIGHTER • WEIGHT MANAGEMENT • VEGAN/VEGETARIAN

30-MINUTE

SERVES 4
Prep time: 10 minutes
Cook time: 20 minutes

1 tablespoon olive oil

2 leeks, white and green parts, cleaned and chopped

2 teaspoons minced garlic

3 cups fresh watercress

3 cups chopped fresh kale

2 tablespoons chopped fresh parsley

4 cups sodium-free vegetable stock

Juice and zest of 1 lemon

1 cup coconut milk

Sea salt, for seasoning

Freshly ground black pepper, for seasoning

Watercress has a unique peppery taste. Similar to the other members of the mustard family, watercress grows in fresh water and is often sold with the roots still attached. It's rich in iodine, iron, calcium, and folic acid as well as vitamins A and C. This dark green, robust vegetable is also very high in phytonutrients and antioxidants, making it a wonderful anti-inflammatory.

1. Heat the olive oil in a medium stockpot over medium-high heat.

2. Add the leeks and garlic and sauté for about 4 minutes, until tender.

3. Stir in the watercress, kale, and parsley and sauté 1 minute.

4. Stir in the vegetable stock, lemon juice, and lemon zest and bring the soup to a boil.

5. Reduce the heat to low and simmer for 15 minutes.

6. Purée the soup with an immersion blender or a food processor until smooth.

7. Return the soup to the stockpot and stir in the coconut milk.

8. Season with salt and pepper.

FERTILITY BOOST TIP: Add 1 cup chopped broccoli to boost the amount of folic acid. Broccoli will add 26 milligrams folic acid per serving. The addition won't affect the taste of the soup, because both kale and watercress have extremely assertive flavors.

PER SERVING Calories: 238; Total fat: 20g; Saturated fat: 15g; Carbs: 16g; Fiber: 4g; Protein: 5g; Sodium: 133mg

SUMMER VEGETABLE MILLET SOUP

FERTILITY BOOST • INFLAMMATION FIGHTER • WEIGHT MANAGEMENT • VEGAN/VEGETARIAN

ONE-POT

SERVES 8
Prep time: 10 minutes
Cook time: 40 minutes

1 tablespoon olive oil

1 sweet onion, chopped

1 tablespoon
minced garlic

1 red bell pepper,
chopped

2 carrots, chopped

6 cups sodium-free
vegetable stock

1 cup green beans, cut
into 1-inch pieces

1 cup cooked millet

Sea salt, for seasoning

Freshly ground black
pepper, for seasoning

The millet is stirred in right at the end of the cooking time so that it doesn't break up or get mushy. Make sure the cooked millet is al dente before you stir it in. Millet is a great source of copper, manganese, phosphorus, and magnesium, and help can reduce the risk of diabetes and heart disease.

1. Heat the olive oil in a large stockpot over medium-high heat.

2. Add the onion and garlic and sauté until for about 3 minutes, until translucent.

3. Stir in the red bell pepper and carrots and sauté for 3 minutes.

4. Add the stock and bring the soup to a boil.

5. Reduce the heat to low and simmer for about 30 minutes, until the vegetables are tender.

6. Stir in the green beans and millet and simmer 4 minutes more.

7. Season with salt and pepper.

VARIATION TIP: Quinoa can be used instead of millet to give the soup more of a nutritional boost. The macronutrients in both ingredients are very similar, although quinoa has slightly less total carbs and more fiber. It also contains more vitamin A, vitamin E, and folate.

PER SERVING Calories: 109; Total fat: 2g; Saturated fat: 0g; Carbs: 17g; Fiber: 4g; Protein: 3g; Sodium: 104mg

TURKEY-CAULIFLOWER CHOWDER

INFLAMMATION FIGHTER • WEIGHT MANAGEMENT

ONE-POT
BULK COOK

SERVES 8
Prep time: 10 minutes
Cook time: 30 minutes

1 tablespoon olive oil

1 sweet onion, chopped

2 teaspoons minced garlic

8 cups sodium-free
chicken stock
(or turkey stock)

4 cups cooked turkey
meat, dark or white

1 sweet potato, diced

½ head cauliflower,
cut into florets

½ cup coconut milk

Sea salt, for seasoning

Freshly ground black
pepper, for seasoning

Chowder is a creamy soup filled with a variety of vegetables and chunks of tender meat or fish. In this dish, turkey, sweet potato, and cauliflower are the stars. Sweet potatoes contain phytonutrients such as polyacetylenes, anthocyanins, and beta-carotene, along with vitamins A, C, and K; potassium; and blood-sugar-stabilizing fiber.

1. Heat the olive oil in a large stockpot over medium-high heat.

2. Add the onion and garlic and sauté for 5 minutes.

3. Add the stock, turkey meat, and sweet potato and bring the soup to a boil.

4. Reduce the heat to low and simmer for about 20 minutes, until the vegetables are tender.

5. Stir in the cauliflower and simmer for about 5 minutes, until the cauliflower is tender but still firm.

6. Stir the coconut milk.

7. Season with sea salt and pepper.

BULK COOKING TIP: Freeze the soup in a large plastic freezer bag rather than a container. Be sure to squeeze all the air out of the bag once it's filled. Then seal the bag and lay it flat on a baking sheet to freeze. This will create an easy-to-store meal that takes up very little room.

PER SERVING Calories: 199; Total fat: 8g; Saturated fat: 4g; Carbs: 9g; Fiber: 2g; Protein: 24g; Sodium: 97mg

KALE-PEAR SOUP

FERTILITY BOOST • WEIGHT MANAGEMENT

30-MINUTE

SERVES 4
Prep time: 5 minutes
Cook time: 20 minutes

1 tablespoon olive oil

½ sweet onion, chopped

1 teaspoon minced garlic

1 teaspoon grated
fresh ginger

4 cups sodium-free
chicken stock

6 cups chopped kale

2 pears, peeled, cored,
and chopped

½ cup low-fat plain
yogurt, divided

Sea salt, for seasoning

Freshly ground black
pepper, for seasoning

2 tablespoons roasted
pumpkin seeds

Recipe garnishes should be much more than just decorative; they need to add a nutritional punch. The pumpkin seeds in this soup are delicious and offer a light, finishing crunch. The seeds are also a fabulous source of the mineral zinc, essential for healthy egg development and the cell division in the early stages of pregnancy.

1. Heat the olive oil in a large stockpot over medium-high heat.

2. Add the onion, garlic, and ginger and sauté about 3 minutes, until softened.

3. Add the stock, kale, and pears and bring the soup to a boil.

4. Reduce the heat to low and simmer for 15 minutes.

5. Transfer the soup to a blender and purée until smooth.

6. Transfer the soup back to the pot and stir in ¼ cup of the yogurt.

7. Season with salt and pepper.

8. Serve topped with remaining yogurt and the pumpkin seeds.

INFLAMMATION-FIGHTING TIP: Leave the skin on the pears. The skin has roughly four times the phenolic phytonutrients than the fruit's flesh. Phytonutrients contain antioxidant anti-inflammatory flavonoids, an important part of a PCOS diet.

PER SERVING Calories: 210; Total fat: 6g; Saturated fat: 1g; Carbs: 31g; Fiber: 6g; Protein: 8g; Sodium: 97mg

WILD RICE PEACH SALAD

INFLAMMATION FIGHTER • WEIGHT MANAGEMENT • VEGAN/ VEGETARIAN

30-MINUTE

SERVES 4
Prep time: 15 minutes

4 cups finely chopped kale

1 red bell pepper, chopped

½ cup cooked wild rice

2 peaches, pitted
and chopped

½ cup prepared raspberry
or balsamic dressing

2 tablespoons
almonds, chopped

Wild rice is a wonderful chewy, nutty tasting addition to cold salads that can be made ahead and stored in the refrigerator in a sealed container for up to 3 or 4 days. You can substitute regular brown rice or quinoa instead if you have those on hand. The wonderful thing about salads is that experimentation can create lovely combinations that will delight the whole family.

1. In a medium bowl, toss together the kale, red bell pepper, wild rice, and peaches with the dressing until well coated.

2. Top the salad with almonds and serve.

FERTILITY BOOST TIP: Use fresh strawberries instead of peaches in this salad, about 2 cups of halved berries. Berries are extremely high in antioxidants, which can help protect eggs from aging and damage.

PER SERVING Calories: 215; Total fat: 13g; Saturated fat: 2g; Carbs: 23g; Fiber: 4g; Protein: 5g; Sodium: 90mg

GREEK CHICKPEA SALAD

INFLAMMATION FIGHTER • VEGAN/VEGETARIAN

30-MINUTE
NO COOK
ONE-POT

SERVES 4
Prep time: 15 minutes

2 cups spinach

1 cup sodium-free
canned chickpeas

1 English cucumber,
chopped

1 yellow bell
pepper, chopped

1 cup cherry
tomatoes, halved

½ red onion, chopped

½ cup prepared
balsamic dressing

What would a Greek salad be without juicy chunks of cucumber? Cucumber is mostly water, but it's also packed with antioxidants and phytonutrients. Cucumbers are a spectacular source of vitamin C, manganese, beta-carotene, cucurbitacin, flavonoids, and lignans.

1. In a medium bowl, toss together the spinach, chickpeas, cucumber, yellow bell pepper, cherry tomatoes, and onion.

2. Add the dressing and toss the salad until well coated.

FERTILITY BOOST TIP: Add 1 cup of white navy beans or kidney beans to increase the iron content in this salad. Adequate iron levels in the body ensure that healthy eggs are produced in ovulation. Beans are also high in protein and fiber, which can help with weight-management goals.

PER SERVING Calories: 265; Total fat: 25g; Saturated fat: 3g; Carbs: 19g; Fiber: 6g; Protein: 7g; Sodium: 226mg

CRUNCHY ASPARAGUS-CRANBERRY SALAD

INFLAMMATION FIGHTER • WEIGHT MANAGEMENT • VEGETARIAN

30-MINUTE
NO COOK
ONE-POT

SERVES 4
Prep time: 20 minutes

20 asparagus stalks, cut into ribbons with a vegetable peeler

2 pears, cored and chopped

½ cup dried cranberries

½ cup sunflower seeds

2 scallions, white and green parts, chopped

2 tablespoons apple cider vinegar

1 tablespoon raw honey

1 tablespoon fresh thyme, chopped

Part of the crunch in this beautiful salad comes from the addition of sunflower seeds. Look for roasted unsalted seeds to avoid the extra sodium. Sunflower seeds are ideal for fighting inflammation because they contain zinc, magnesium, and vitamins B_2 and B_6. Vitamin B_6 deficiency can increase the effect of inflammation in the body, so add a couple extra tablespoons of sunflower seeds as a pretty garnish.

1. In a large bowl, toss together the asparagus ribbons, pears, cranberries, sunflower seeds, and scallions.

2. Stir together the apple cider vinegar, honey, and thyme in a small bowl.

3. Add the dressing to the vegetables and toss to combine.

COOKING TIP: Cut off the woody ends of the asparagus, about 1 inch, to ensure a lovely tender ribbon. If you have a mandolin, use it to create perfectly thin ribbons.

PER SERVING Calories: 139; Total fat: 3g; Saturated fat: 0g; Carbs: 24g; Fiber: 6g; Protein: 4g; Sodium: 6mg

CITRUS ROASTED CAULIFLOWER SALAD

FERTILITY BOOST • INFLAMMATION FIGHTER • WEIGHT MANAGEMENT • VEGAN/VEGETARIAN

5-INGREDIENT
30-MINUTE

SERVES 4
Prep time: 10 minutes
Cook time: 20 minutes

1 cauliflower head, cut into florets

¼ cup olive oil, divided

½ teaspoon minced garlic

Sea salt, for seasoning

Freshly ground black pepper, for seasoning

¼ cup pecan halves

2 tablespoons chopped fresh parsley

Juice of 1 lemon

Roasted cauliflower has an almost nutty flavor that is enhanced by the addition of buttery smooth pecans. Pecans come from the hickory tree. For hundreds of years they were a staple food for indigenous people. This tree nut was prized for its disease- and inflammation-fighting nutrients such as vitamin E, omega-3 fatty acid, ellagic acid, oleic acid, lutein, and beta-carotene.

1. Preheat the oven to 425°F.

2. Line a baking sheet with parchment.

3. In a large bowl, toss together the cauliflower, 1 tablespoon olive oil, and garlic until coated.

4. Spread the florets on the baking sheet and season lightly with salt and pepper.

5. Roast until the cauliflower is caramelized, about 20 minutes.

6. Transfer the cauliflower back to the bowl and add the pecans and parsley. Toss to combine.

7. In a small bowl, whisk together the remaining olive oil and lemon juice and add the salad.

8. Toss and serve.

VARIATION TIP: For a little color and sweetness, you can add diced sweet potato or carrot to the cauliflower and roast the vegetables together. The dish will have an extra inflammation-fighting boost of beta-carotene.

PER SERVING Calories: 159; Total fat: 14g; Saturated fat: 2g; Carbs: 11g; Fiber: 4g; Protein: 2g; Sodium: 83mg

THAI TAHINI SLAW

FERTILITY BOOST • INFLAMMATION FIGHTER • WEIGHT MANAGEMENT • VEGAN/VEGETARIAN

30-MINUTE
NO COOK

SERVES 4
Prep time: 20 minutes

1 head cabbage, shredded

2 carrots, shredded

1 scallion, white and green parts, chopped

½ cup roasted peanuts, chopped

2 tablespoons chopped fresh cilantro

½ cup Tahini Peanut Sauce (page 188)

This colorful and flavorful dish is not your grandma's coleslaw. The dressing is nutty, hot, and sweet. Chopped peanuts add a unique texture to the slaw. If possible, make the slaw the day before. The extra time will allow the flavors to better meld.

1. In a large bowl, toss together the cabbage, carrots, scallion, peanuts, and cilantro.

2. Add the dressing and toss to combine.

LEFTOVER TIP: If you have a very large cabbage and end up with extra, you can use the cabbage for soups, side dishes, casseroles, or another fiber-packed salad. You can also use a small Napa cabbage instead of green cabbage.

PER SERVING Calories: 247; Total fat: 16g; Saturated fat: 2g; Carbs: 19g; Fiber: 7g; Protein: 9g; Sodium: 70mg

CHERRY AND BRUSSELS SPROUTS SALAD

FERTILITY BOOST • VEGETARIAN

30-MINUTE
NO COOK

SERVES 4
Prep time: 25 minutes

FOR THE DRESSING

¼ cup olive oil

2 tablespoons apple cider vinegar

1 tablespoon raw honey

2 teaspoons Dijon mustard

½ teaspoon fresh thyme, chopped

Sea salt, for seasoning

Freshly ground black pepper, for seasoning

FOR THE SALAD

5 cups Brussels sprouts, shredded

1 cup pitted cherries, halved

2 scallions, white and green parts, chopped

½ avocado, chopped

½ cup hazelnuts, chopped

The hazelnuts in the dish aren't just for taste; they bring significant nutritional benefits due to their impressive quantities of fiber, monounsaturated fatty acids, vitamin E, and folate. These nutrients help support fertility and boost the immune system. For a truly sublime flavor, toast the hazelnuts in a 300°F oven for about 15 minutes before you chop them up.

FOR THE DRESSING

1. In a small bowl, whisk together the olive oil, apple cider vinegar, honey, mustard, and thyme.

2. Season with salt and pepper.

FOR THE SALAD

1. In a large bowl, toss together the Brussels sprouts, cherries, and scallions.

2. Add the dressing and toss to coat.

3. Serve topped with avocado and hazelnuts.

INFLAMMATION-FIGHTING TIP: Add a cup of blueberries along with the cherries for extra color and an extra boost of antioxidants. Blueberries are high in polyphenols, a chemical substance that triggers antioxidant activity in the body.

PER SERVING Calories: 307; Total fat: 22g; Saturated fat: 3g; Carbs: 22g; Fiber: 8g; Protein: 6g; Sodium: 118mg

BROILED PLUM SPINACH SALAD

FERTILITY BOOST • INFLAMMATION FIGHTER • VEGAN/VEGETARIAN

30-MINUTE

SERVES 4
Prep time: 15 minutes
Cook time: 3 minutes

4 plums, halved and pitted

¼ cup plus 1 teaspoon olive oil, divided

⅛ teaspoon ground cinnamon

2 tablespoons balsamic vinegar

1 tablespoon chopped fresh basil

Freshly ground black pepper, for seasoning

4 cups spinach

½ English cucumber, diced

½ cup shredded fennel

¼ cup cashews, chopped

Broiled or barbecued fruit has a sublime caramelized sweetness that explodes in your mouth. The lovely texture combines perfectly with both tender greens and crunchy nuts. Plums are in season from about May to August, so it's best to prepare this dish during that time of year. Plums are an excellent source of vitamins C and K, as well as fiber, copper, and potassium. The fruit can also increase iron absorption in the body, which is crucial for fertility.

1. Preheat the oven to broil.

2. Place the plum halves cut side up on a pie plate and brush them lightly with 1 teaspoon olive oil. Sprinkle the tops with cinnamon and broil until the fruit is lightly caramelized, about 3 minutes.

3. Remove the fruit from the oven and chop.

4. In a medium bowl, whisk together the remaining olive oil, balsamic vinegar, and basil and season with pepper.

5. Add the spinach, cucumber, and fennel to the bowl and toss to coat.

6. Arrange the salads on two plates and top with broiled plums and cashews.

FERTILITY BOOST TIP: Add 2 cups of lightly blanched asparagus cut into 1-inch pieces, to increase the amount of folic acid in the salad. Four asparagus stalks contain 90 milligrams folic acid along with plenty of vitamins A, C, and K.

PER SERVING Calories: 205; Total fat: 17g; Saturated fat: 3g; Carbs: 14g; Fiber: 3g; Protein: 3g; Sodium: 32mg

SPINACH-PECAN SALAD WITH HARDBOILED EGGS

FERTILITY BOOST • INFLAMMATION FIGHTER • WEIGHT MANAGEMENT • VEGETARIAN

5-INGREDIENT
30-MINUTE
ONE-POT
BULK COOK

SERVES 4
Prep time: 10 minutes

8 cups baby spinach

4 hardboiled eggs, cut into eighths

1 pear, cored and diced

½ cup prepared poppy seed dressing

½ cup pecan pieces

Sometimes simple is best when it comes to creating a filling salad for lunch or a light dinner. Darky leafy greens, crunchy nuts, rich eggs, and a sweet pear are the perfect combination of textures and flavors. The poppy seed dressing will add calcium, iron, and zinc to the dish, which supports healthy ovulation and regulates hormone levels.

1. Arrange the spinach on four plates and top with egg wedges and pear.

2. Drizzle the dressing over the salads and top each with pecans.

BULK COOKING TIP: If you need a pretty salad for a community gathering or large dinner, this recipe will fit the bill. Instead of arranging the salads on individual plates, toss the spinach, pears, dressing and pecans in a large bowl all together and then top with egg wedges.

PER SERVING Calories: 382; Total fat: 24g; Saturated fat: 6g; Carbs: 24g; Fiber: 3g; Protein: 9g; Sodium: 504mg

SALMON-ARUGULA SALAD

FERTILITY BOOST • INFLAMMATION FIGHTER • WEIGHT MANAGEMENT

5-INGREDIENT
30-MINUTE

SERVES 4
Prep time: 10 minutes

8 cups baby arugula

1 cup shredded fennel

8 radishes, thinly sliced

½ cup prepared vinaigrette

4 (5-ounce) cooked
salmon fillets

Adding salmon to your salad is a healthy choice for a PCOS diet plan. Salmon is an oily fish and an excellent source of omega-3 fatty acids, a powerful anti-inflammatory. It also helps regulate reproductive hormones and improve blood flow to the uterus and ovaries.

1. Place the arugula, fennel, and radishes in a bowl and toss the vegetables with the vinaigrette.

2. Arrange the salad on four plates and top each with salmon.

COOKING TIP: The salmon can be made several days ahead and kept in the refrigerator in a sealed container or sealed plastic bag. You can also use leftover salmon or any other fish leftover from dinner to top this lovely salad.

PER SERVING Calories: 219; Total fat: 11g; Saturated fat: 2g; Carbs: 5g; Fiber: 2g; Protein: 22g; Sodium: 314mg

Millet-Stuffed Tomatoes, *page 63*

FOUR

EASY APPETIZERS AND SIDES

TOMATO-PLUM BRUSCHETTA

INFLAMMATION FIGHTER • WEIGHT MANAGEMENT • VEGAN/VEGETARIAN

30-MINUTE
ONE POT
NO COOK

SERVES 4
Prep time: 20 minutes

2 tomatoes, seeded
and diced

2 plums, pitted and diced

½ yellow bell
pepper, chopped

1 scallion, sliced thinly

1 tablespoon lime juice

1 teaspoon olive oil

1 teaspoon chopped
fresh basil

Pinch sea salt

4 slices sprouted grain
bread, lightly toasted

Tomatoes and plums may seem like an unusual pairing, but the sweetness and texture of each of these fruits are delicious together. Any type of plum will do, but deep dark black plums look glorious with the red and yellow vegetables and green herbs. Black plums are high in vitamin A, vitamin C, and potassium, which can reduce inflammation.

1. In a medium bowl, stir together the tomatoes, plums, yellow bell pepper, scallion, lime juice, olive oil, and basil.

2. Season with salt.

3. Spoon the mixture onto the bread and serve.

INGREDIENT TIP: Sprouted grain products are available in most grocery stores, usually in the freezer section. For this bread, the wheat grains are first sprouted and then ground into flour. The process creates a bread with fewer carbs, gluten, and fat, but more protein than regular wheat bread.

PER SERVING Calories: 108; Total fat: 2g; Saturated fat: 1g; Carbs: 19g; Fiber: 4g; Protein: 4g; Sodium: 167mg

WHITE BEAN-STUFFED MUSHROOMS

INFLAMMATION FIGHTER • VEGAN/VEGETARIAN

SERVES 4

Prep time: 15 minutes
Cook time: 20 minutes

12 white mushrooms, stemmed

1 tablespoon olive oil

½ cup canned white beans

¼ cup sun-dried tomatoes, chopped

1 scallion, white and green parts, chopped

1 teaspoon chopped fresh basil

⅛ teaspoon minced garlic

Sea salt, for seasoning

Freshly ground black pepper, for seasoning

½ cup almond flour

This colorful mixture with its red and green flecks also makes a great spread for wraps and sandwiches. White beans are low on the glycemic index and won't raise your blood sugar. They're also a good source of protein and soluble fiber. Look for canned white beans or navy beans with no added sodium.

1. Preheat the oven to 400°F.

2. Line a baking sheet or pie plate with parchment paper and set aside.

3. Toss the mushroom caps with the olive oil and lay them hollow side down on the baking sheet.

4. Bake until softened and lightly browned, about 10 minutes.

5. Remove the caps from the oven and flip them over.

6. In a small bowl, mash the beans together with the sun-dried tomatoes, scallion, basil, and garlic.

7. Season the mixture with salt and pepper and scoop it evenly into the mushroom caps.

8. Sprinkle the caps with almond flour and bake in the oven until golden brown and hot, about 10 minutes.

FERTILITY BOOST TIP: Use cooked split peas instead of white beans to add extra fiber. This can help regulate blood sugar and balance hormones. Cooked split peas contain about 17 grams of fiber per cup, which adds about 2 grams per serving.

PER SERVING Calories: 184; Total fat: 10g; Saturated fat: 1g; Carbs: 17g; Fiber: 5g; Protein: 9g; Sodium: 136mg

CRISPY ZUCCHINI FRIES

INFLAMMATION FIGHTER • WEIGHT MANAGEMENT • VEGETARIAN

5-INGREDIENT

SERVES 4
Prep time: 15 minutes
Cook time: 20 minutes

1 pound zucchini

½ cup cornstarch

2 eggs

2 cups almond flour

1 teaspoon garlic powder

Sea salt, for seasoning

Freshly ground black pepper, for seasoning

Zucchini isn't a firm vegetable and doesn't contain a lot of natural sugar, so it won't crisp or caramelize on its own without a fatty coating. Almond flour works well as a coating because it browns beautifully, and the delicate nutty flavor doesn't overpower the taste of the zucchini. Almond flour has no glycemic impact on blood sugar and is packed with anti-inflammatory components. Almonds are also a fantastic source of omega-3 fatty acids, protein, magnesium, and calcium.

1. Preheat the oven to 400°F and line a baking sheet with parchment.

2. Cut the zucchini into 4-inch long and ½-inch wide batons and set aside.

3. Arrange three medium bowls in a row on a clean work surface and place the cornstarch in the first, beat the eggs in the second, and stir together the almond flour and garlic powder in the third.

4. Dredge the zucchini batons in the cornstarch, then the eggs, and then the almond flour mixture. Be sure to thoroughly coat the vegetables.

5. Place the breaded fries on the baking sheet. When all the zucchini is breaded, season the fries lightly with salt and pepper.

6. Bake the fries until golden brown, 18 to 20 minutes.

INGREDIENT TIP: Look for medium zucchini with a glossy skin free of soft spots and cracks. Larger zucchini can be bitter, soft, and too seedy to cut into batons. You can use either color of zucchini, yellow or green.

PER SERVING Calories: 197; Total fat: 9g; Saturated fat: 1g; Carbs: 20g; Fiber: 3g; Protein: 7g; Sodium: 102mg

BAKED ONION RINGS

INFLAMMATION FIGHTER • WEIGHT MANAGEMENT • VEGAN/VEGETARIAN

5-INGREDIENT

SERVES 4
Prep time: 20 minutes
Cook time: 20 minutes

Olive oil spray

1½ cups gluten-free flour blend

1 cup sodium-free vegetable stock

2 tablespoons arrowroot flour

2 cups almond flour

2 large sweet onions, peeled and cut into ½-inch slices

Whether your onion rings are baked or fried, they need an even layer of batter or breading to create a crispy texture. To achieve this, use arrowroot flour. This powdery ingredient is made from the ground-up roots of the arrowroot plant. Arrowroot flour is high in omega-3 fatty acids, calcium, and potassium and it is gluten-free.

1. Preheat the oven to 425°F.

2. Lightly spray a baking sheet. Set aside.

3. In a medium bowl, whisk together the flour, stock, and arrowroot flour until the batter is smooth.

4. Place the almond flour in a medium bowl.

5. Separate the onions into individual rings and select about 40 good-size ones. Reserve the remaining onion in the refrigerator for another recipe.

6. Dip the rings into the batter, coating them completely. Shake off the excess and then dredge the rings in the almond flour, completely coating the vegetable.

7. Place the coated onion rings on the baking sheet and repeat until all the rings are done.

8. Lightly spray the breaded onion rings with olive oil spray. Bake until crispy and golden, 18 to 20 minutes, turning once halfway through the cooking time.

9. Serve immediately.

INGREDIENT TIP: If available, use Vidalia onions. The variety is milder and sweeter than regular yellow or white onions. Vidalia onions are a great source of vitamin C, an antioxidant, and chromium, a mineral that can enhance the action of insulin.

PER SERVING Calories: 220; Total fat: 8g; Saturated fat: 1g; Carbs: 32g; Fiber: 8g; Protein: 7g; Sodium: 12mg

MUSHROOM QUESADILLAS

FERTILITY BOOST • WEIGHT MANAGEMENT • VEGAN/VEGETARIAN

30-MINUTE

SERVES 4

Prep time: 15 minutes
Cook time: 12 minutes

4 (8-inch) sprouted grain tortillas

1 tablespoon olive oil

3 cups cremini mushrooms, sliced

1 cup finely shredded kale

¼ cup prepared basil pesto

¼ cup sun-dried tomatoes, chopped

1 scallion, white and green parts, thinly sliced

Cremini mushrooms look similar in shape to button mushrooms, but with a slightly darker shade of brown. They are usually right next to each other in the produce section at the grocery store. Cremini mushrooms are loaded with vitamin B_2, an important nutrient for normal thyroid function and healthy metabolism. Sufficient vitamin B_2 can reduce the risk of issues associated with excessive testosterone and androgen such as acne and thinning hair.

1. Preheat the oven to broil.

2. Place the tortillas on a baking sheet and toast in the oven until crisp, about 1 minute.

3. Remove from the oven and set aside.

4. Place a large skillet over medium-high heat and add the olive oil.

5. Sauté the mushrooms until they are tender and lightly caramelized, about 5 minutes.

6. Add the kale and sauté until wilted, about 4 minutes. Remove the skillet from the heat and set aside.

7. Spread 1 tablespoon of pesto on each tortilla.

8. Divide the mushroom mixture evenly between the tortillas, spreading it out to about 1 inch from the edges.

9. Sprinkle each tortilla with sun-dried tomatoes and scallion.

10. Place the baking sheet back in the oven and broil until the topping is heated through and caramelized.

11. Cut the tortillas into four pieces each and serve.

INFLAMMATION-FIGHTING TIP: Top the quesadillas with ¼ cup of chopped artichoke hearts. Artichoke hearts are a rich source of phytonutrients, more than traditional antioxidant superfoods such as blueberries and dark chocolate.

PER SERVING Calories: 230; Total fat: 13g; Saturated fat: 3g; Carbs: 20g; Fiber: 3g; Protein: 8g; Sodium: 278mg

ZUCCHINI-WRAPPED VEGETABLE ROLLS

INFLAMMATION FIGHTER • WEIGHT MANAGEMENT • VEGAN/VEGETARIAN

30-MINUTE

SERVES 4
Prep time: 25 minutes
Cook time: 30 seconds

½ cup finely shredded red cabbage

1 carrot, shredded

1 red bell pepper, julienned

1 scallion, both green and white parts, julienned

2 tablespoons chopped fresh cilantro

2 teaspoons olive oil

1 teaspoon sesame seeds

¼ teaspoon ground cumin

¼ teaspoon ground coriander

2 zucchini, sliced into very thin lengthwise strips with a vegetable peeler

Zucchini grows prolifically and to enormous sizes, so if you're growing it in your garden, you're probably always looking for recipes to make a dent in the bounty. Using zucchini for these colorful crunchy rolls is inspired. The snack might become a family favorite. Zucchini is very high in beta-carotene, zeaxanthin, and lutein, which are potent antioxidants. Leave the skin on the zucchini when you peel the vegetable. It will firm the edges on the thin strips and support the shape. Plus, the skin is packed with antioxidants.

1. In a medium bowl, toss together the cabbage, carrot, red bell pepper, scallion, cilantro, olive oil, sesame seeds, cumin, and coriander until well mixed. Set aside.

2. Place a medium saucepan filled with water on high heat and bring to a boil.

3. Lightly blanch 8 perfect strips of zucchini in boiling water for 30 seconds and then lay the strips on paper towels to completely dry them.

4. Evenly divide the vegetable filling between the zucchini strips, placing the filling close to one end of the strip.

5. Roll up the strips around the filling and secure with a wooden toothpick.

6. Repeat with each strip and serve 2 per person.

SUBSTITUTION TIP: You can also use English cucumbers instead of zucchini if you prefer, and you do not have to blanch them. Blot the cucumber dry before rolling up the veggies. Make sure you choose cucumbers that do not have excessive seeds, or the rolls could fall apart.

PER SERVING Calories: 60; Total fat: 3g; Saturated fat: 0g; Carbs: 8g; Fiber: 3g; Protein: 2g; Sodium: 24mg

MILLET-STUFFED TOMATOES

FERTILITY BOOST • INFLAMMATION FIGHTER • WEIGHT MANAGEMENT • VEGAN/VEGETARIAN

5-INGREDIENT

SERVES 4
Prep time: 15 minutes
plus 30 minutes
draining time
Cook time: 25 minutes

4 large tomatoes

½ teaspoon sea salt

1 tablespoon olive oil

1 sweet onion, chopped

1 cup finely chopped
cauliflower

1 cup cooked millet

¼ cup pine nuts

Pinch freshly ground
black pepper

The pine nuts in this recipe add a lovely earthy flavor to the filling. They're often used for baking or in basil pesto recipes. But they also provide a satisfying crunch to any type of dish. This golden kernel is actually the seed of the pine tree, not a nut. Pine nuts are packed with inflammation-busting antioxidants, iron, protein, magnesium, and healthy monounsaturated fats that are crucial for balancing hormones.

1. Cut the tops off the tomatoes and discard.

2. Scoop out the insides of the tomatoes leaving the shell intact.

3. Sprinkle the inside of the shells with the salt, and turn the tomatoes upside down on paper towels for 30 minutes to drain the juices.

4. Place the tomatoes hollow side up in a small baking dish.

5. Preheat the oven to 350°F.

6. Place a large skillet over medium-high heat and add the olive oil.

CONTINUED

7. Sauté the onion until softened, about 3 minutes.

8. Add the cauliflower and sauté, about 2 minutes.

9. Remove the skillet from the heat and stir in the millet, pine nuts, and pepper and mix well.

10. Spoon the millet mixture evenly between the tomatoes.

11. Bake until the filling is heated through and the tomatoes are softened, about 20 minutes.

SUBSTITUTION TIP: Try using baked sweet potatoes, acorn squash, or zucchini as the containers to hold this fiber- and nutrient-packed filling. After you've scooped out the vegetables, save the extra flesh for other recipes such as soups or side dishes.

PER SERVING Calories: 244; Total fat: 10g; Saturated fat: 1g; Carbs: 30g; Fiber: 8g; Protein: 8g; Sodium: 207mg

SIMPLE RATATOUILLE

FERTILITY BOOST • WEIGHT MANAGEMENT • VEGAN/VEGETARIAN

ONE-POT
BULK COOK

SERVES 4
Prep time: 15 minutes
Cook time: 55 minutes

1 tablespoon olive oil

1 red onion, diced

1 tablespoon
minced garlic

½ eggplant, peeled and
diced into 1-inch chunks

1 yellow bell pepper, diced

1 zucchini, diced

1 (15-ounce) can
sodium-free diced tomato

¼ cup sodium-free
vegetable stock

Pinch red pepper flakes

Sea salt, for seasoning

Freshly ground black
pepper, for seasoning

Hormone balance is a huge concern for women with PCOS. Eating foods that stabilize the hormones is crucial, such as fruits and vegetables. Too much estrogen can increase the chance of heart disease, intensify PMS symptoms, and cause depression. Vegetable-packed ratatouille gives you a range of colors, including greens, red, and yellow, and loads of antioxidants. Several of the ingredients in ratatouille are high in vitamin C, which can increase progesterone production and create a better balance with estrogen.

1. Place a large saucepan over medium-high heat and add the olive oil.

2. Sauté the onion and garlic until softened, about 3 minutes.

3. Add the eggplant, yellow bell pepper, and zucchini and sauté 5 minutes more.

4. Stir in the diced tomatoes, vegetable stock, and red pepper flakes and bring the mixture to a boil.

5. Reduce the heat to low and simmer until thick, stirring occasionally, about 45 minutes.

6. Season with salt and pepper.

BULK COOKING TIP: Ratatouille is a perfect recipe to freeze because the vegetables are not meant to retain their shape. The texture is similar to a very chunky sauce. Make sure you allow the ratatouille to come to room temperature before freezing, to avoid ice crystals and freezer burn.

PER SERVING Calories: 92; Total fat: 4g; Saturated fat: 1g; Carbs: 13g; Fiber: 4g; Protein: 3g; Sodium: 75mg

SPRING VEGETABLE MÉLANGE

INFLAMMATION FIGHTER • WEIGHT MANAGEMENT • VEGAN/VEGETARIAN

30-MINUTE
ONE-POT

SERVES 4
Prep time: 15 minutes
Cook time: 15 minutes

1 tablespoon olive oil

1 teaspoon minced garlic

2 carrots, sliced

¼ head cauliflower,
cut into small florets

¼ head broccoli,
cut into small florets

1 cup green beans,
cut into 1-inch pieces

1 red bell pepper,
cut into strips

1 yellow zucchini,
cut into thin rounds

2 teaspoons fresh
thyme, chopped

Sea salt, for seasoning

Freshly ground black
pepper, for seasoning

Everyone should have one tried-and-true vegetable dish that goes with different meat, poultry, or fish dishes; even better if it's delicious and filling enough to stand on its own. What could be easier or more beautiful than a mélange of assorted seasonal vegetables? This assortment has orange, white, yellow, red, and several shades of green, so you know there is a broad range of antioxidants on the plate, including beta-carotene, lutein, chlorophyll, and lycopene.

1. Place a large skillet over medium-high heat and add the olive oil.

2. Sauté the garlic until softened, about 2 minutes.

3. Add the carrots and sauté for 3 minutes.

4. Stir in the cauliflower and broccoli and sauté for 4 minutes.

5. Add the green beans, red bell pepper, zucchini, and thyme. Sauté the vegetables until they are tender crisp, about 5 minutes.

6. Season the vegetables with salt and pepper and serve.

FERTILITY BOOST TIP: Olive oil is part of a healthy diet and addresses some issues associated with PCOS. This monounsaturated fat can help decrease inflammation in the body and increase insulin sensitivity. Inflammation can impede healthy ovulation and the development of the embryo.

PER SERVING Calories: 90; Total fat: 4g; Saturated fat: 1g; Carbs: 13g; Fiber: 4g; Protein: 3g; Sodium: 107mg

ROASTED CAULIFLOWER
AND CELERY ROOT

FERTILITY BOOST • INFLAMMATION FIGHTER • WEIGHT MANAGEMENT • VEGETARIAN

30-MINUTE

SERVES 4
Prep time: 10 minutes
Cook time: 20 minutes

½ head cauliflower, cut into florets

1 celery root, peeled and diced

1 tablespoon olive oil

Sea salt, for seasoning

Freshly ground black pepper, for seasoning

¼ cup coconut milk

1 tablespoon raw honey

Juice from ½ lemon

½ teaspoon ground nutmeg

Celery root or celeriac is exactly what it sounds like—the root of the celery plant. Although you can find this bulbous root vegetable year-round, it's best in the late fall, winter, and early spring. Celery root is rich in antioxidants, calcium, fiber, and vitamins B_6, C, and K. This underutilized and visually unattractive ingredient can help stabilize blood sugar and boost immunity.

1. Preheat the oven to 400°F.

2. Line a baking sheet with parchment paper and set aside.

3. In a large bowl, toss together the cauliflower, celery root, and oil until the vegetables are coated.

4. Season the vegetables lightly with salt and pepper.

5. Transfer the vegetables to the baking sheet and roast in the oven until very tender and lightly caramelized, about 20 minutes.

6. Remove the vegetables from the oven and transfer to a bowl.

7. Stir in the coconut milk, honey, lemon juice, and nutmeg and mash until fluffy.

FERTILITY BOOST TIP: Although celery root adds an interesting flavor and texture to this dish, you can also use cauliflower alone to create a lovely mashed side. Cauliflower is an exceptional source of choline—a blood sugar–regulating fiber—and folate. Use the entire cauliflower head instead of half if you're omitting the celery root.

PER SERVING Calories: 123; Total fat: 7g; Saturated fat: 4g; Carbs: 14g; Fiber: 3g; Protein: 2g; Sodium: 149mg

MUSHROOM, CELERY, AND WILD RICE PILAF

INFLAMMATION FIGHTER • WEIGHT MANAGEMENT • VEGAN/VEGETARIAN

30-MINUTE
ONE-POT

SERVES 4
Prep time: 10 minutes
Cook time: 20 minutes

1 tablespoon olive oil

2 teaspoons minced garlic

2 cups sliced mushroom

2 celery stalks, chopped

1½ cups cooked quinoa

½ cup cooked wild rice

Sea salt, for seasoning

Freshly ground black pepper, for seasoning

2 scallions, white and green parts, chopped

If you are looking for an elegant dish, this gorgeous pilaf will do the trick. The dark-colored grains and chewy texture of the wild rice make for an intriguing mix. The celery, quinoa, and wild rice are high in fiber, so blood sugar levels won't spike after you enjoy the pilaf. Try adding other vegetables or other types of onions for delicious variations.

1. Place a large skillet over medium-high heat and add the olive oil.

2. Sauté the garlic until softened, about 2 minutes.

3. Stir in the mushrooms and celery and sauté until the vegetables are lightly caramelized and tender, about 10 minutes.

4. Stir in the quinoa and wild rice and sauté until warmed through, about 6 minutes.

5. Season with salt and pepper and serve topped with scallions.

INFLAMMATION-FIGHTING TIP: Olive oil is always a healthy choice for cooking. It contains 138 milligrams of omega-3 fatty acid per tablespoon, which is a spectacular inflammation fighter. Walnut oil also works beautifully with the other ingredients in this recipe; it will boost the omega-3 amounts by about 1,320 milligrams.

PER SERVING Calories: 179; Total fat: 5g; Saturated fat: 1g; Carbs: 25g; Fiber: 4g; Protein: 7g; Sodium: 77mg

ZUCCHINI PANCAKES

FERTILITY BOOST • WEIGHT MANAGEMENT • VEGAN/VEGETARIAN

30-MINUTE

SERVES 4
Prep time: 10 minutes
Cook time: 16 minutes

½ pound zucchini, shredded then wrapped in a dish towel and squeezed to remove excess water

1 cup almond flour

1 carrot, shredded

¼ sweet onion, chopped

2 eggs

2 teaspoons lemon zest

1 teaspoon minced garlic

½ teaspoon baking powder

⅛ teaspoon freshly ground black pepper

Sea salt, for seasoning

¼ cup olive oil, for frying

Pancakes or latkes are what you call these tender, lightly browned patties. The carrot in this recipe brings more structure to the mixture because it is firmer than zucchini. Serve the pancakes with sautéed apples or pears, plus a scoop of plain low-fat Greek yogurt for a sublime meal. The yogurt adds hormone-balancing fat and the fruit brings a plethora of anti-inflammatory antioxidants.

1. In a large bowl, combine the zucchini, almond flour, carrot, onion, eggs, lemon zest, garlic, baking powder, and pepper until well mixed.

2. Season the mixture with salt.

3. Place a large skillet over medium-high heat and add the olive oil.

4. Scoop the zucchini mixture, about ¼ cup, into the skillet and press down with a fork to create flat pancakes. About four pancakes can fit easily in a skillet.

5. Cook the pancakes until golden brown and lightly crispy around the edges, flipping once, about 8 minutes in total.

6. Transfer the pancakes to paper towels and repeat with the remaining batter.

INFLAMMATION-FIGHTING TIP: Shred half a sweet potato and add it to the zucchini mixture. Sweet potato is packed with vitamin A, a potent antioxidant, as well as beta-carotene.

PER SERVING Calories: 94; Total fat: 6g; Saturated fat: 1g; Carbs: 7g; Fiber: 2g; Protein: 5g; Sodium: 107mg

SAUTÉED CHILI CABBAGE

FERTILITY BOOST • INFLAMMATION FIGHTER • WEIGHT MANAGEMENT • VEGAN/VEGETARIAN

30-MINUTE
ONE-POT
BULK COOK

SERVES 4
Prep time: 10 minutes
Cook time: 20 minutes

2 teaspoons olive oil

1 teaspoon sesame oil

2 tablespoons grated
fresh ginger

2 teaspoons minced garlic

1 head cabbage, finely
shredded

3 tablespoons
coconut aminos

1 teaspoon chili sauce
such as sambal oelek

Freshly ground black
pepper, for seasoning

You can find many varieties of chili sauce on your grocery shelves. Choose your favorite or discover a new gem for this recipe. Chiles have a double whammy of fighting inflammation and supporting fertility. They also stimulate the endorphins to reduce stress and can improve blood flow to the reproductive organs.

1. Place a large skillet over medium-high heat and add the olive oil and sesame oil.

2. Sauté the ginger and garlic until softened, about 3 minutes.

3. Stir in the cabbage and sauté until lightly caramelized and tender, about 15 minutes.

4. Stir in the coconut aminos and chili sauce.

5. Season with pepper and serve.

BULK COOKING TIP: This dish is a wonderful addition to a potluck dinner or neighborhood barbecue. When doubling the recipe, use 4 tablespoons of coconut aminos and about 1½ teaspoons of chili sauce instead of doubling the amount of both ingredients. This dish should not be frozen.

PER SERVING Calories: 104; Total fat: 4g; Saturated fat: 1g; Carbs: 14g; Fiber: 5g; Protein: 4g; Sodium: 645mg

CREAMED LEEKS AND SPINACH

FERTILITY BOOST • INFLAMMATION FIGHTER

30-MINUTE
ONE-POT

SERVES 4
Prep time: 10 minutes
Cook time: 20 minutes

1 tablespoon olive oil

3 leeks, white and green parts, sliced and cleaned

¼ cup sodium-free chicken stock

4 cups spinach

½ cup coconut milk

½ teaspoon ground nutmeg

Sea salt, for seasoning

Freshly ground black pepper, for seasoning

Leeks are often bypassed for the more familiar onion, which is a shame because this incredible ingredient has a marvelous texture and taste. When preparing the leeks, cut off the tougher green parts near the very top. Leeks have folate in both the white and green sections and are a superb source of kaempferol (a flavonoid), copper, vitamin K, and manganese, so they are an excellent choice to support fertility.

1. Place a large skillet over medium-high heat and add the olive oil.

2. Sauté the leeks until they are tender and lightly caramelized, about 10 minutes.

3. Stir in the chicken stock and spinach and sauté until the spinach is wilted, about 4 minutes.

4. Stir in the coconut milk and cook, stirring, until the coconut mixture is creamy and hot, about 3 minutes.

5. Stir in the nutmeg and season with salt and pepper.

FERTILITY BOOST TIP: Try collard greens instead of spinach in this dish. Collard greens are a little more robust than spinach, so you'll need to double the cook time to 8 minutes in step 3. They provide 177 milligrams of folic acid per serving compared with spinach, which has 26 milligrams.

PER SERVING Calories: 148; Total fat: 11g; Saturated fat: 7g; Carbs: 12g; Fiber: 3g; Protein: 3g; Sodium: 100mg

PISTACHIO RICE PILAF

INFLAMMATION FIGHTER • WEIGHT MANAGEMENT

5-INGREDIENT
ONE-POT

SERVES 4
Prep time: 10 minutes
Cook time: 30 minutes

1 tablespoon olive oil

½ sweet onion, chopped

½ cup brown rice

1 cup sodium-free
chicken stock

1 cup finely chopped
cauliflower

Sea salt, for seasoning

Freshly ground black
pepper, for seasoning

¼ cup chopped pistachios

Pistachios are a little pricey, but the luxurious nut is well worth it. To save a little time, you can buy shelled pistachios. To save a little money, buy them whole and shell them yourself. Regardless, you certainly don't want to skimp on the nuts; they add a distinctive crunch and healthy omega-3 fatty acids. Pistachios are also high in protein, fiber, and antioxidants such as carotenes and vitamin E.

1. Place a medium saucepan over medium heat and add the olive oil.

2. Sauté the onion until softened, about 3 minutes.

3. Add the rice and sauté 2 minutes.

4. Add the chicken stock and bring the rice to a boil. Reduce the heat to low and simmer, covered, until the liquid is absorbed, about 20 minutes.

5. Stir in the cauliflower, about 5 minutes, or until tender when pierced with a fork.

6. When the cauliflower rice is cooked, season with salt and pepper.

7. Stir in the pistachios.

FERTILITY BOOST TIP: Add a chopped red bell pepper along with the cauliflower. Bell peppers are high in vitamin C and can help the body absorb the iron in the brown rice. The mineral is crucial for fertility.

PER SERVING Calories: 159; Total fat: 6g; Saturated fat: 1g; Carbs: 21g; Fiber: 4g; Protein: 5g; Sodium: 312mg

SESAME GREEN BEANS

FERTILITY BOOST • INFLAMMATION FIGHTER • WEIGHT MANAGEMENT • VEGAN/VEGETARIAN

5-INGREDIENT
30-MINUTE

SERVES 4
Prep time: 10 minutes
Cook time: 12 minutes

1 pound green
beans, trimmed

½ red bell pepper,
finely chopped

1 tablespoon
sesame seeds

1 teaspoon sesame oil

Pinch red pepper flakes

Sea salt, for seasoning

With the right choices you can create a spectacular dish with only a handful of ingredients. In this recipe, the bright al dente beans, a scattering of red bell pepper, the rich sesame flavor, and a hint of heat create culinary perfection. Green beans are a great source of nutrients that are both inflammation fighting and fertility boosting. They also contain antioxidants, including neoxanthin, lutein, and chlorophyll, as well as fiber, folate, and vitamins K and C. Look for slender uniformly green beans with no rust-colored areas or withered ends.

1. Preheat the oven to 400°F.

2. Line a baking sheet with parchment and set aside.

3. Place a medium saucepan filled with water on high heat and bring to a boil.

4. Blanch the green beans in the boiling water until tender crisp, about 2 minutes.

5. Drain and transfer the beans to a medium bowl.

6. Add the red bell pepper, sesame seeds, sesame oil, and red pepper flakes to the bowl and toss to combine.

7. Transfer to the baking sheet and roast for 10 minutes.

8. Season with salt and serve.

INFLAMMATION-FIGHTING TIP: Substitute walnut oil and chopped walnuts for the sesame products. Walnut oil is very high in omega-3 fatty acids, which can help reduce inflammation in the body. Look for black walnuts whenever possible; the variety does not have the bitterness found in other walnuts.

PER SERVING Calories: 63; Total fat: 2g; Saturated fat: 0g; Carbs: 9g; Fiber: 5g; Protein: 3g; Sodium: 66mg

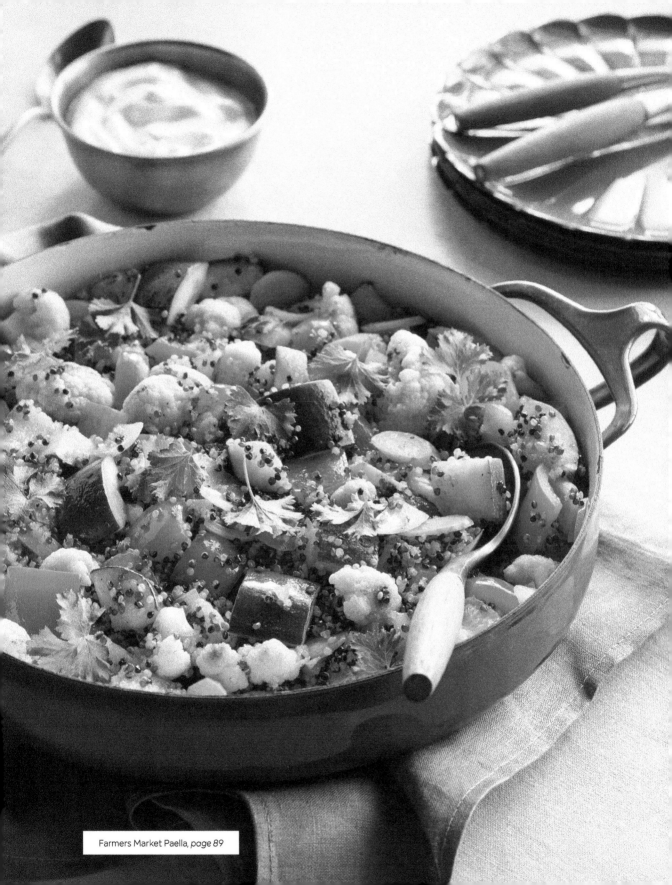

Farmers Market Paella, *page 89*

VEGAN AND VEGETARIAN MAINS

QUINOA-EDAMAME BOWL

FERTILITY BOOST · INFLAMMATION FIGHTER · WEIGHT MANAGEMENT · VEGAN/VEGETARIAN

5-INGREDIENT
30-MINUTE
ONE-POT
BULK COOK

SERVES 3
Prep time: 10 minutes

2 cups cooked quinoa

2 cups shredded bok choy

1 cup shelled edamame

1 red bell pepper, diced

2 tablespoons finely chopped fresh cilantro

Sea salt, for seasoning

Freshly ground black pepper, for seasoning

Edamame is one of those ingredients that used to be very difficult to find but now because of its popularity as a nutritional superfood, you can find it in nearly every grocery store's freezer section. Edamame are immature soybeans, often sold in the pods. They are a wonderful source of protein, comparable with the quality found in milk and eggs. The protein in these tasty little beans also contains a unique peptide that can help improve blood sugar levels and boost immune function.

1. In a large bowl, toss together the quinoa, bok choy, edamame, red pepper, and cilantro.

2. Season with salt and pepper and serve.

BULK COOKING TIP: If you plan to double or triple this recipe, watch the amount of cilantro. In large amounts this herb can be very strong. Start with the original amount and add the chopped herb by teaspoons until the desired flavor is reached.

PER SERVING Calories: 353; Total fat: 9g; Saturated fat: 1g; Carbs: 47g; Fiber: 11g; Protein: 20g; Sodium: 46mg

SOUTHWEST SWEET POTATOES

FERTILITY BOOST • INFLAMMATION FIGHTER • WEIGHT MANAGEMENT • VEGAN/VEGETARIAN

5-INGREDIENT

SERVES 4
Prep time: 10 minutes
Cook time: 30 minutes

4 sweet potatoes, cut
into quarters

1 tablespoon olive oil

Sea salt, for seasoning

Freshly ground black
pepper, for seasoning

2 cups cooked sodium-
free canned lentils

1 cup prepared salsa

1 avocado, diced

2 tablespoons chopped
fresh cilantro

The cilantro garnish for this dish is not just decorative; it is also packed with vitamin K and many phytonutrients. Cilantro can help regulate blood sugar and is often referred to as the antidiabetic plant in areas of Asia. If you like the flavor of this pungent herb, increase the amount in the recipe to 3 tablespoons. For an interesting preparation and presentation, you can use baked sweet potatoes. Simply scoop them out and add the cooked sweet potato to the other ingredients before spooning the filling back into the hollowed spud.

1. Preheat the oven to 400°F.

2. Line a baking sheet with foil and set aside.

3. In a medium bowl, toss the sweet potato and olive oil until the vegetables are well coated.

4. Spread the sweet potatoes on the baking sheet and season lightly with salt and pepper.

5. Bake until tender, about 30 minutes.

CONTINUED

6. Remove from the oven and set aside.

7. While the sweet potatoes are cooking, place a medium skillet over medium heat and add the lentils and salsa.

8. Stir until heated through, about 5 minutes.

9. Arrange four quarters of sweet potato on each plate and top with a generous spoon of the lentil mixture. Divide the avocado between the plates.

10. Serve topped with cilantro.

INFLAMMATION-FIGHTING TIP: Include ½ cup to 1 cup chopped roasted red bell pepper in this dish for its inflammation fighting capabilities. Bell peppers are a stellar source of anti-oxidants such as vitamin C, luteolin, beta-carotene, and quercetin, which neutralize inflammation-causing free radicals.

PER SERVING Calories: 347; Total fat: 10g; Saturated fat: 2g; Carbs: 50g; Fiber: 20g; Protein: 13g; Sodium: 345mg

CAULIFLOWER-TOMATO STEW

FERTILITY BOOST • INFLAMMATION FIGHTER • WEIGHT MANAGEMENT • VEGAN/VEGETARIAN

**5-INGREDIENT
ONE-POT**

SERVES 4
Prep time: 10 minutes
Cook time: 30 minutes

2 tablespoons olive oil

1 sweet onion, chopped

1 head cauliflower, cut
into small florets

1 (28-ounce) can
sodium-free diced
tomatoes

2 cups cooked
sodium-free black beans

4 cups chopped
Swiss chard

Sea salt, for seasoning

Freshly ground black
pepper, for seasoning

The Swiss chard in this stew adds a lovely earthy flavor.
The dark green leaves are extremely high in vitamin B_6,
a crucial nutrient for fertility. Vitamin B_6 can help prevent
PMS and morning sickness symptoms as well as balance
hormones such as progesterone and estrogen. Swiss
chard is also effective for regulating blood sugar and
supporting cardiovascular health.

1. Heat the olive oil in a large saucepan over
medium-high heat.

2. Add the onion and sauté until softened, about
3 minutes.

3. Add the cauliflower and sauté for 5 minutes more.

4. Stir in the tomatoes and black beans and bring the
mixture to a boil.

5. Reduce the heat and simmer, stirring frequently,
until the cauliflower is tender, about 15 minutes.

6. Remove from the heat and stir in the Swiss chard.

7. Let the stew stand until the chard is wilted, about
4 minutes.

8. Season with salt and pepper.

VARIATION TIP: Any dark leafy green would be fabulous, so use
whatever you have handy in the refrigerator, or whatever suits your
palate. Try kale, spinach, beet greens, or collard greens in the same
amount as the chard.

PER SERVING Calories: 250; Total fat: 7g; Saturated fat: 1g; Carbs: 35g; Fiber: 15g;
Protein: 13g; Sodium: 133mg

QUICK CHICKPEA-AVOCADO TOAST

FERTILITY BOOST • INFLAMMATION FIGHTER • VEGAN/VEGETARIAN

5-INGREDIENT
30-MINUTE
NO COOK

SERVES 4
Prep time: 10 minutes

2 cups canned
sodium-free chickpeas

1 tablespoon olive oil

Sea salt, for seasoning

Freshly ground black
pepper, for seasoning

8 slices sprouted
grain bread

2 tomatoes, thinly sliced

1 avocado, pitted
and diced

1 cup alfalfa sprouts

Some days simply scream out for an easy and quick meal. Toast is perfect solution because it allows for an infinite choice of toppings. The sprouts in this recipe make the dish festive, plus they add a healthy dose of vitamin K and phytoestrogens. This combination can help regulate estrogen and minimize PMS symptoms. Alfalfa sprouts have also been found to lower blood glucose levels and fight inflammation in the body.

1. Place the chickpeas and olive oil in a blender and pulse until thick, but with chunks.

2. Season the mixture lightly with salt and pepper.

3. Toast the bread and place the slices on a clean work surface.

4. Spread the chickpeas on the bread and top each with tomatoes, avocado, and sprouts.

5. Serve two slices per person.

WEIGHT MANAGEMENT TIP: Use only half of an avocado to cut down on calories, total fat, and carbs. The dish will still be delicious and filling.

PER SERVING Calories: 418; Total fat: 18g; Saturated fat: 3g; Carbs: 49g; Fiber: 17g; Protein: 16g; Sodium: 203mg

MISO-ROASTED EGGPLANT AND ZUCCHINI

INFLAMMATION FIGHTER • WEIGHT MANAGEMENT • VEGAN/VEGETARIAN

5-INGREDIENT
ONE-PAN
BULK COOK

SERVES 4
Prep time: 10 minutes
Cook time: 30 minutes

1 large eggplant, cut into 1-inch slices

2 zucchini, cut into quarters lengthwise

1 tablespoon olive oil

¼ cup white miso paste

1 tablespoon sesame seeds

2 scallions, white and green parts, chopped

Miso may be a new ingredient in your culinary repertoire, but it is readily available in nearly every major grocery store, usually in the organic section. Miso is a paste made with fermented soybeans and is packed with probiotics and anti-inflammatory compounds. Miso helps support the gut-friendly bacteria in your body, making it easier to absorb nutrients from food and helping reduce inflammation.

1. Preheat the oven to 400°F.

2. Line a baking sheet with foil and set aside.

3. Arrange the eggplant and zucchini on the baking sheet and brush the vegetables with oil and the miso paste.

4. Roast until tender and lightly browned, about 30 minutes.

5. Serve the vegetables topped with sesame seeds and scallions.

BULK COOKING TIP: Only the size of your oven and number of baking sheets you possess will limit how much of this tasty dish you can prepare. Arrange the finished vegetables on a colorful platter for a lovely presentation.

PER SERVING Calories: 105; Total fat: 5g; Saturated fat: 1g; Carbs: 13g; Fiber: 6g; Protein: 3g; Sodium: 60mg

SPICY FALAFEL

FERTILITY BOOST · INFLAMMATION FIGHTER · WEIGHT MANAGEMENT · VEGETARIAN

30-MINUTE

SERVES 4
Prep time: 20 minutes
Cook time: 10 minutes

1½ cups canned
sodium-free chickpeas

¼ cup almond flour

1 scallion, chopped

½ teaspoon ground cumin

Pinch sea salt

1 egg

1 tablespoon olive oil

2 (6-inch) sprouted grain
pitas, halved crosswise

1 tomato, diced

½ avocado, diced

¼ cup low-fat plain
Greek yogurt

Chickpeas are the classic choice for the base of these savory patties, but fava beans are also used in some recipes. Chickpeas are an ideal PCOS diet–friendly ingredient because they help regulate blood sugar and create a slow-release form of energy. Chickpeas are also an excellent source of fiber, folate, vitamins C and E, and beta-carotene, which support fertility and the immune system.

1. Place the chickpeas in a blender and pulse until coarsely mashed.

2. Add the almond flour, scallion, cumin, and salt and pulse to combine.

3. Add the egg and pulse until the bean mixture holds together. Add a little water if the mixture is too crumbly.

4. Shape the mixture into four patties, about ½-inch thick.

5. Place a large skillet over medium-high heat and add the olive oil.

6. Cook the patties until they are lightly browned, turning once, about 5 minutes per side.

7. Blot the patties with paper towels to remove any excess oil.

8. Stuff one patty into each pita half and top with the tomato, avocado, and yogurt.

9. Serve one pita half per person.

INFLAMMATION-FIGHTING TIP: Falafel can be spiced with an assortment of flavors such as coriander, cinnamon, and turmeric. Add ½ teaspoon of ground turmeric to the recipe; this pungent spice contains curcumin, a compound that can reduce inflammation in the body.

PER SERVING Calories: 298; Total fat: 11g; Saturated fat: 2g; Carbs: 39g; Fiber: 10g; Protein: 13g; Sodium: 218mg

OAT RISOTTO WITH LEEKS AND MUSHROOMS

FERTILITY BOOST • INFLAMMATION FIGHTER • WEIGHT MANAGEMENT • VEGAN/VEGETARIAN

ONE-POT

SERVES 4
Prep time: 15 minutes
Cook time: 25 minutes

1 tablespoon olive oil

2 leeks, white and green parts, chopped

2 cups sliced white mushrooms

2 teaspoons garlic, minced

2 cups sodium-free vegetable stock

1 cup quick-cooking oats

1 cup shredded spinach

1 tablespoon chopped fresh basil

Sea salt, for seasoning

Fresh ground black pepper, for seasoning

Oats are a superb breakfast choice and equally delicious and nutritious as a savory meal choice. This unassuming little grain is gluten-free and loaded with antioxidants, fiber, minerals, and vitamins. Oats are linked to weight loss, reduced risk of cardiovascular disease, and can lower blood sugar. Oats are also an excellent source of manganese, phosphorus, magnesium, copper, iron, and zinc.

1. Place a large skillet over medium-high heat and add the olive oil.

2. Sauté the leeks, mushrooms, and garlic until lightly caramelized and tender, about 10 minutes.

3. Stir in the vegetable stock, oats, and spinach.

4. Reduce the heat to medium and cook, stirring, until most of the liquid is absorbed and the oats are creamy, about 15 minutes.

5. Stir in the basil and season the risotto with salt and pepper.

INGREDIENT TIP: To add a little extra flavor to this dish include 1 tablespoon nutritional yeast. The yeast has a cheesy, nutty flavor that works well in many recipes. It's packed with magnesium, protein, zinc, and B vitamins. You can find this ingredient in the organic section of most grocery stores.

PER SERVING Calories: 155; Total fat: 5g; Saturated fat: 1g; Carbs: 22g; Fiber: 4g; Protein: 6g; Sodium: 78mg

SOUTHWEST MILLET
AND BLACK BEAN BOWL

FERTILITY BOOST • INFLAMMATION FIGHTER • WEIGHT MANAGEMENT • VEGETARIAN

30-MINUTE
ONE-POT

SERVES 4
Prep time: 10 minutes
Cook time: 20 minutes

1 tablespoon coconut oil

1 sweet onion, chopped

½ jalapeño pepper, minced

1 cup finely chopped cauliflower

1 cup cooked millet

1 cup canned sodium-free black beans, rinsed

1 cup cherry tomatoes, halved

¼ cup chopped fresh cilantro

Some cooks avoid mixing black beans with other ingredients because if not drained properly, the beans can give the dish a grayish hue. But don't let that discourage you. These glossy black legumes are as high in antioxidants as colorful vegetables and fruits. Black beans contain a generous amount of flavonoids, including quercetin, malvidin, and kaempferol, along with many others. They can boost fertility because they are also high in iron, protein, and folate.

1. Place a large saucepan over medium-high heat and add the coconut oil.

2. Add the onion and jalapeño and sauté until softened, about 3 minutes.

3. Stir in the cauliflower and sauté until tender, about 5 minutes.

4. Add the millet and cook, stirring occasionally until just heated through, about 10 minutes.

5. Remove from the heat and stir in the black beans and cherry tomatoes.

6. Serve topped with cilantro.

LEFTOVER TIP: Scoop the leftovers into a sprouted grain pita bread or wrap for an energy-packed lunch or snack. You can also top a fresh green salad with a couple spoonfuls of the mixture and a sliced chicken breast.

PER SERVING Calories: 245; Total fat: 8g; Saturated fat: 1g; Carbs: 34g; Fiber: 9g; Protein: 9g; Sodium: 34mg

MIXED VEGETABLE LETTUCE WRAPS

INFLAMMATION FIGHTER · WEIGHT MANAGEMENT · VEGAN/VEGETARIAN

30-MINUTE
ONE-POT

SERVES 4
Prep time: 20 minutes
Cook time: 7 minutes

1 tablespoon coconut oil

½ sweet onion, chopped

1 teaspoon minced garlic

1 carrot, shredded

1 yellow zucchini, shredded

1 cup green beans, cut into ½-inch pieces

1 cup sodium-free canned red lentils

Juice and zest of 1 lime

1 tablespoon chopped cilantro

8 large Boston lettuce leaves

Boston lettuce is often the most delicate green available in produce section at the grocery store. It's often grown in a hydroponic greenhouse. You'll find it sealed in a small plastic bag and sold with the roots still attached. You should be able to get eight respectably sized leaves from one head of lettuce. Use the remaining leaves in a salad. Boston lettuce is extremely high in chromium, a mineral that can regulate blood sugar levels and help control food cravings.

1. Place a large skillet over medium-high heat and add the oil.

2. Add the onion and garlic and sauté until softened, about 3 minutes.

3. Stir in the carrot, zucchini, and green beans and sauté 4 minutes.

4. Stir in the lentils, lime juice, lime zest, and cilantro.

5. Spoon the filling into the lettuce leaves and serve.

INFLAMMATION TIP: Top these wraps with sunflower seeds for a huge boost in vitamin E, copper, and B vitamins. The tiny seeds are also an excellent source of omega-3 fatty acids and add a marvelous crunch to this dish.

PER SERVING Calories: 198; Total fat: 8g; Saturated fat: 4g; Carbs: 24g; Fiber: 9g; Protein: 9g; Sodium: 26mg

COCONUT VEGETABLE STEW

INFLAMMATION FIGHTER • VEGAN/VEGETARIAN

ONE-POT

SERVES 4
Prep time: 20 minutes
Cook time: 30 minutes

2 garlic cloves

1-inch piece fresh
ginger, peeled

½ jalapeño
pepper, chopped

Juice and zest of 1 lime

1½ cups coconut milk

½ cup sodium-free
vegetable stock

2 cups shredded cabbage

1 cup shredded carrot

1 cup small
cauliflower florets

1 red bell pepper, sliced
into thin strips

The spiciness of this stew should be no surprise; the added heat is a perfect complement to the coconut. If you are a coconut enthusiast, stir in ½ cup of shredded unsweetened coconut into the stew at the end. Or top the dish with lightly toasted coconut. Shred your own fresh coconut for a real treat and strong flavor.

1. Pured the garlic, ginger, jalapeño, pepper, lime juice, and lime zest in a blender until smooth. Set aside.

2. Place a large saucepan over medium-high heat and add the coconut milk and vegetable stock.

3. Bring the liquid to a boil and stir in the garlic mixture.

4. Reduce the heat to low and simmer until the flavors mellow and the liquid is reduced by a third, 20 to 25 minutes.

5. Stir in the cabbage, carrot, cauliflower, and red bell pepper.

6. Simmer until the vegetables are tender, about 3 minutes.

WEIGHT MANAGEMENT TIP: If you have a taste for heat, use the entire jalapeño pepper instead of half. Jalapeños are rich in vitamin C as well as a phytonutrient called capsaicin, which can increase the feeling of fullness. Capsaicin is a thermogenic agent, which increases the metabolism.

PER SERVING Calories: 250; Total fat: 20g; Saturated fat: 19g; Carbs: 14g; Fiber: 5g; Protein: 6g; Sodium: 147mg

NAVY BEAN SHEPHERD'S PIE

INFLAMMATION FIGHTER • WEIGHT MANAGEMENT • VEGAN/VEGETARIAN

BULK COOK

SERVES 4
Prep time: 15 minutes
Cook time: 45 minutes

2 sweet potatoes, peeled and cut into chunks

¼ cup coconut milk

Sea salt, for seasoning

Freshly ground black pepper, for seasoning

1 tablespoon olive oil

1 sweet onion, chopped

2 teaspoons minced garlic

2 cups chopped cauliflower

2 cups sodium-free canned navy beans

2 large tomatoes, chopped

½ cup frozen green peas

2 teaspoons dried thyme

The origins of shepherd's pie stems from sheep herders who prepared the dish with lamb. This vegetarian take doesn't compromise on flavor or nutritional value. The pie is flavored with fresh thyme, an herb known for its healing powers. Thyme can reduce the risk of diabetes and insulin resistance, as well as support a healthy immune system. This delicate fragrant herb is a wonderful source of fiber, iron, copper, vitamin A, and vitamin C.

1. Preheat the oven to 350°F.

2. Place the sweet potatoes in a large saucepan filled with water and bring them to a boil.

3. Reduce the heat and simmer until the potatoes are fork tender, about 15 minutes.

4. Drain the potatoes and mash them with the coconut milk.

5. Season the mashed sweet potatoes with salt and pepper and set aside.

6. While the sweet potatoes are cooking, place a large skillet over medium-high heat and add the olive oil.

7. Add the onion and garlic and sauté until softened, about 3 minutes.

CONTINUED

8. Stir in the cauliflower and sauté until the vegetables are tender, about 10 minutes.

9. Stir in the navy beans, tomatoes, peas, and thyme and transfer the mixture to a 9-by-9 casserole dish.

10. Top the vegetable mixture with the mashed sweet potatoes, and bake the casserole until it is hot and the vegetables are very tender, about 30 minutes.

FERTILITY BOOST TIP: Add 3 cups of mushrooms to boost the amount of vitamin D in the casserole. Vitamin D can also help increase the number of mature follicles in the ovaries and regulate the menstrual cycle.

PER SERVING Calories: 289; Total fat: 8g; Saturated fat: 4g; Carbs: 43g; Fiber: 13g; Protein: 10g; Sodium: 55mg

FARMERS MARKET PAELLA

INFLAMMATION FIGHTER • WEIGHT MANAGEMENT • VEGAN/VEGETARIAN

ONE-POT

SERVES 4
Prep time: 15 minutes
Cook time: 25 minutes

1 tablespoon olive oil

1 sweet onion, chopped

2 teaspoons minced garlic

1 zucchini, diced

1 carrot, thinly sliced

1 red bell pepper, diced

1 cup small
cauliflower florets

2 cups cooked quinoa

Sea salt, for seasoning

Freshly ground black
pepper, for seasoning

3 tablespoons fresh
parsley, chopped

Parsley, with its lovely color and earthy flavor, is more than just a garnish for this colorful dish. The herb is loaded with anti-inflammatory agents such as flavonoids and vitamin C. It also has a volatile oil called eugenol, which is a powerful antioxidant capable of ridding the body of harmful toxins. Parsley can also boost the immune system and improve digestion. In some cultures, the herb is chewed after meals.

1. Place a large skillet over medium-high heat and add the olive oil.

2. Add the onion and garlic and sauté for about 3 minutes, until softened.

3. Stir in the zucchini, carrot, red pepper, and cauliflower and sauté until the vegetables are tender crisp, about 10 minutes.

4. Stir in the quinoa and sauté until just heated through, about 10 minutes.

5. Season with salt and pepper.

6. Serve topped with parsley.

FERTILITY BOOST TIP: Top the paella with a couple tablespoons of Greek yogurt for a creamy finish. Yogurt is a high in vitamin D, which can help the follicles in your ovaries mature. It's also a great source of protein and calcium.

PER SERVING Calories: 229; Total fat: 6g; Saturated fat: 1g; Carbs: 35g; Fiber: 7g; Protein: 9g; Sodium: 95mg

BEAN-STUFFED ZUCCHINI

FERTILITY BOOST • INFLAMMATION FIGHTER • WEIGHT MANAGEMENT • VEGAN/VEGETARIAN

BULK COOK

SERVES 4
Prep time: 10 minutes
Cook time: 25 minutes

4 zucchini, cut in half lengthwise, seeds scooped out to form hollow containers

2 tablespoons olive oil, divided

½ sweet onion, chopped

2 teaspoons minced garlic

2 cups cooked navy beans, rinsed and drained

1 cup shredded spinach

½ cup cooked millet

1 carrot, grated

¼ cup hazelnuts, chopped

Sea salt, for seasoning

Freshly ground black pepper, for seasoning

Meal planning is not always enjoyable, especially when you're trying to maintain a specific nutritional point of view, but eating always should be. These stuffed zucchini boats are fun and nutritious. There is something whimsical about hollowing out the zucchini and spooning in the colorful, textured filling. The best part of the meal besides its wonderful flavor is the nutritional value.

1. Preheat the oven to 400°F.

2. Line a baking sheet with parchment. Place the zucchini halves on the sheet, hollow side up, and brush the cut side with 1 tablespoon olive oil.

3. Bake the zucchini in the oven until softened, about 6 minutes.

4. While the zucchini are cooking, place a medium skillet over medium-high heat and add the remaining olive oil.

5. Add the onion and garlic and sauté until softened, about 3 minutes.

6. Stir in the navy beans, spinach, millet, carrot, and hazelnuts.

7. Sauté for 3 minutes more.

8. Season the filling with salt and pepper.

9. Remove the zucchini from the oven and spoon the filling evenly into the hollows.

10. Place the zucchini back in the oven and bake 10 minutes more.

SUBSTITUTION TIP: Cooked quinoa and brown rice are also great choices for this filling.

PER SERVING Calories: 306; Total fat: 12g; Saturated fat: 2g; Carbs: 34g; Fiber: 10g; Protein: 11g; Sodium: 99mg

CHILLED ASIAN VEGGIE NOODLES

INFLAMMATION FIGHTER • WEIGHT MANAGEMENT • VEGETARIAN

30-MINUTE

SERVES 2
Prep time: 15 minutes
Cook time: 6 minutes

FOR THE SAUCE

1 tablespoon olive oil

¼ cup rice vinegar

2 tablespoons
coconut aminos

2 teaspoons grated
fresh ginger

1 teaspoon raw honey

½ teaspoon minced garlic

FOR THE NOODLES

2 zucchini, spiralized or
cut into ribbons with
a vegetable peeler

1 carrot, spiralized or cut
into ribbons with a
vegetable peeler

1 cup bean sprouts

1 red bell pepper,
julienned

1 tablespoon
sesame seeds

When you see the colorful vegetables and taste the exciting Asian-influenced sauce, this dish will quickly fold into your weekly cooking regimen. Bean sprouts are soaked and sprouted legumes. The process removes the enzyme inhibitor from the legume so the sprouts can develop. Bean sprouts help promote good digestion and better mineral absorption in the body. They're also high in essential fatty acids, vitamins A, B-complex, C, and E, as well as fiber.

FOR THE SAUCE

1. In a small bowl, whisk together the olive oil, rice vinegar, coconut aminos, ginger, honey, and garlic until well blended.

2. Set aside.

FOR THE NOODLES

1. Place a large skillet over medium heat and add the sauce.

2. Sauté the zucchini, carrot, bean sprouts, and red bell pepper until tender crisp, about 5 minutes.

3. Add the sauce and toss to coat. Sauté 1 minute more.

4. Serve topped with sesame seeds.

FERTILITY BOOST: Substitute blackstrap molasses for honey to get more nutrients. The rich ingredient is high in antioxidants, iron, B vitamins, and calcium. Molasses is low on the glycemic index and contains chromium, which can help regulate blood sugar.

PER SERVING Calories: 296; Total fat: 17g; Saturated fat: 3g; Carbs: 27g; Fiber: 7g; Protein: 9g; Sodium: 899mg

HEARTY VEGETABLE-BEAN STEW

FERTILITY BOOST · INFLAMMATION FIGHTER · WEIGHT MANAGEMENT · VEGAN/VEGETARIAN

BULK COOK

SERVES 4
Prep time: 15 minutes
Cook time: 30 minutes

1 tablespoon olive oil

1 sweet onion, chopped

1 tablespoon minced garlic

2 cups sodium-free vegetable stock, divided

1 (15-ounce) can sodium-free diced tomatoes

3 cups cooked navy beans

1 sweet potato, peeled and diced

1 carrot, diced

2 teaspoons ground cumin

Sea salt, for seasoning

Freshly ground black pepper, for seasoning

2 cups Swiss chard, chopped

You can use pre-ground cumin in the recipe or you can buy whole cumin seeds and grind them yourself. If you plan to self-grind, first toast the seeds in a skillet over low heat for a couple minutes, then place in a clean coffee grinder and pulse. Freshly ground cumin results in a nutty citrus flavor. Cumin is a fantastic source of iron, calcium, manganese, and magnesium. It's also known to be beneficial for fertility and can boost your metabolism.

1. Place a large stock pot over medium-high heat and add the olive oil.

2. Add the onion and garlic and sauté until softened, about 3 minutes.

3. Stir in the vegetable stock, tomatoes, navy beans, sweet potato, carrot, and cumin.

4. Bring to a boil, then reduce heat to low and simmer until the beans and vegetables are very tender, about 20 minutes.

5. Season with salt and pepper.

6. Stir in the chard and let the stew sit for 5 minutes to wilt the greens.

BULK COOKING TIP: Double the stew recipe and freeze the extra portions for a quick and easy meal.

PER SERVING Calories: 246; Total fat: 5g; Saturated fat: 1g; Carbs: 41g; Fiber: 13g; Protein: 10g; Sodium: 290mg

CLASSIC LENTIL DAL

INFLAMMATION FIGHTER • WEIGHT MANAGEMENT • VEGAN/VEGETARIAN

30-MINUTE
ONE-POT
BULK COOK

SERVES 4
Prep time: 5 minutes
Cook time: 25 minutes

1 tablespoon coconut oil

1 sweet onion, chopped

1 tablespoon grated
fresh ginger

2 teaspoons minced garlic

3 tablespoons red
curry paste

1 (15-ounce) can
sodium-free diced
tomatoes

½ cup coconut milk

4 cups cooked lentils

2 cups chopped kale

2 tablespoons chopped
fresh cilantro

Lentils and warm spices are a comfortable, classic combination found in many dishes. In this recipe the lentils retain their shape and the kale adds color and texture, so it's not as soft as a traditional dal. Curry spice is a blend of many inflammation-fighting superstar spices such as turmeric, ginger, cinnamon, and cumin.

1. Place a large saucepan over medium-high heat and add the oil.

2. Add the onion, ginger, and garlic and sauté until softened and fragrant, about 3 minutes.

3. Stir in the red curry paste and sauté 1 minute.

4. Add the tomatoes and coconut milk and bring the sauce to a boil.

5. Reduce the heat to low and simmer 15 minutes.

6. Stir in the lentils and kale and simmer 5 minutes.

7. Serve the curry over brown rice or cauliflower rice topped with cilantro.

BULK COOKING TIP: When doubling this recipe, only use 1 tablespoon of coconut oil to sauté the vegetables. You only need enough to coat the bottom of the pan. Too much oil can create an unpleasant film of fat and extra calories in the finished dish.

PER SERVING Calories: 236; Total fat: 13g; Saturated fat: 10g; Carbs: 22g; Fiber: 6g; Protein: 7g; Sodium: 345mg

QUINOA VEGGIE BURGERS

INFLAMMATION FIGHTER • WEIGHT MANAGEMENT • VEGAN/VEGETARIAN

BULK COOK

SERVES 4
Prep time: 15 minutes,
plus 30 minutes
chilling time
Cook time: 15 minutes

2 teaspoons olive oil

½ sweet onion, chopped

2 teaspoons minced garlic

1 cup cooked quinoa

1 cup canned
sodium-free lentils

½ cup cashews, chopped

½ teaspoon ground cumin

Sea salt, for seasoning

Freshly ground black
pepper, for seasoning

Olive oil spray

The base of these burgers is quinoa, which is a complete protein. The seed is also low on the glycemic index, and packed with antioxidants. Quinoa is high in fiber, omega-3 fatty acids, vitamin E, oleanic acid, and saponins.

1. Place a medium skillet over medium-high heat and add the olive oil.

2. Add the onion and garlic and sauté until softened, about 3 minutes.

3. Transfer the onion and garlic to a food processor and add the quinoa, lentils, cashews, and cumin. Pulse until the mixture holds together. Add a little sodium-free vegetable stock if the mixture is too crumbly.

4. Season the mixture with salt and pepper, divide the mixture into four portions, and form each into a patty about 3 ½ inches in diameter.

5. Place veggie patties in the refrigerator for about 30 minutes to chill.

6. Preheat the oven to broil.

7. Spray the patty on both sides lightly with olive oil spray and place on a baking sheet.

8. Broil for about 5 minutes per side, until the patties are golden and heated through.

9. Serve the burgers with your favorite toppings.

PER SERVING Calories: 240; Total fat: 12g; Saturated fat: 2g; Carbs: 25g; Fiber: 6g; Protein: 10g; Sodium: 134mg

FRIED CAULIFLOWER RICE

FERTILITY BOOST • WEIGHT MANAGEMENT • VEGAN/VEGETARIAN

ONE-POT

SERVES 2
Prep time: 20 minutes
Cook time: 20 minutes

2 teaspoons olive oil

1 teaspoon sesame oil

2 teaspoons grated
fresh ginger

1 teaspoon minced garlic

1 cup sliced mushrooms

1 cup chopped broccoli

1 cup finely
chopped carrot

¼ cup sodium-free
vegetable stock

1 tablespoon
coconut aminos

4 cups finely
chopped cauliflower

Although not quite as firm as the real grain, finely chopped cauliflower prepared the right way makes an excellent rice substitute. Cauliflower contains phytonutrients, which can help reduce the risk of estrogen dominance, a condition that affects many women with PCOS. Cauliflower is exceptionally high in folate, omega-3 fatty acids, choline, and vitamins C, K, and B$_1$, and can also boost fertility.

1. Place a large skillet over medium-high heat and add the olive oil and sesame oil.

2. Add the ginger and garlic and sauté for 3 minutes.

3. Add the mushrooms, broccoli, and carrot and sauté for 5 minutes

4. Stir in the vegetable stock, coconut aminos, and cauliflower.

5. Stir until the cauliflower rice and other vegetables are tender, about 10 minutes.

VARIATION TIP: Although this recipe is vegetarian, the cauliflower and flavorings work well as a base for many other variations of fried rice. You can add chopped shrimp, chicken, or a host of other vegetables.

PER SERVING Calories: 169; Total fat: 8g; Saturated fat: 1g; Carbs: 20g; Fiber: 8g; Protein: 8g; Sodium: 378mg

ZUCCHINI NOODLES WITH ROASTED RED PEPPER SAUCE

FERTILITY BOOST • INFLAMMATION FIGHTER • WEIGHT MANAGEMENT • VEGAN/VEGETARIAN

30-MINUTE
ONE-POT

SERVES 2
Prep time: 15 minutes
Cook time: 15 minutes

2 teaspoons olive oil

1 sweet onion, chopped

2 teaspoons minced garlic

1 cup roasted red bell peppers, chopped

1 carrot, shredded

½ cup tomato, chopped

1 tablespoon balsamic vinegar

¼ cup shredded fresh basil

Pinch red pepper flakes

Sea salt, for seasoning

Freshly ground black pepper, for seasoning

3 zucchini, cut into long noodles with a peeler or spiralized

Pasta dishes can evoke visions of sunlit patios and lots of laughter with family and friends. These feelings of well-being make sense; pasta seems like home for many people. The noodles in this recipe aren't traditional, but they combine nicely with the slightly smoky sauce. Plus, the green noodles covered in the richly hued sauce makes for a striking presentation. If you are a pasta person, you might want to invest in a spiralizer to create a blend of long vegetable noodles for similar recipes.

1. Place a large skillet over medium-high heat and add the olive oil.

2. Sauté the onion and garlic until softened, for about 3 minutes.

3. Stir in the roasted red peppers, carrot, tomato, balsamic vinegar, basil, and red pepper flakes and cook, stirring, until the chunky sauce is piping hot and chunky, 10 to 12 minutes.

4. Season the sauce with salt and pepper.

5. Add the zucchini noodles to the sauce and toss.

COOKING TIP: To roast your own peppers, cut them in half and scoop out the membrane and seeds. Place the lightly oiled red bell peppers on a baking sheet, cut sides down, in a 400°F oven and roast, until lightly charred, about 20 minutes. Place the peppers in a stainless steel bowl and cover tightly with plastic wrap to steam the skins off. Peel the skin off the peppers and slice.

PER SERVING Calories: 147; Total fat: 5g; Saturated fat: 1g; Carbs: 22g; Fiber: 6g; Protein: 6g; Sodium: 175mg

VEGETARIAN SLOPPY JOES

FERTILITY BOOST • INFLAMMATION FIGHTER • WEIGHT MANAGEMENT • VEGAN/VEGETARIAN

ONE-POT
BULK COOK

SERVES 4
Prep time: 10 minutes
Cook time: 30 minutes

1 tablespoon olive oil

1 sweet onion, chopped

2 celery stalks, chopped

1 tablespoon
minced garlic

1 carrot, shredded

1 (15-ounce) can crushed
tomatoes

½ cup sodium-free
vegetable stock

2 tablespoons mild
chili powder

2 cups cooked red lentils

Sea salt, for seasoning

Freshly ground black
pepper, for seasoning

4 sprouted grain buns

Sloppy Joes are messy and fun to eat. In this recipe the texture of the lentils is surprisingly close to ground beef. Many of the other ingredients, such as the celery, onion, tomatoes, and garlic, are in classic meat Sloppy Joe recipes. If you have leftovers or don't want to eat the mixture on buns, it's equally delightful on cauliflower rice or plain brown rice. Both choices would add fertility-boosting nutrients such as choline and fiber to the meal.

1. Place a large saucepan over medium-high heat and add the olive oil.

2. Add the onion, celery, and garlic and sauté until softened, about 4 minutes.

3. Stir in the carrot, tomatoes, stock, and chili powder.

4. Bring the mixture to a boil and then reduce the heat to low and simmer, stirring frequently, until the mixture is thick and the vegetables tender, about 20 minutes.

5. Stir in the lentils and heat for 5 minutes.

6. Season the mixture with salt and pepper.

7. Divide the filling between the buns and serve.

BULK COOKING TIP: Watch the chili powder quantities when doubling this recipe. Be sure to add the extra by teaspoons until you reach the desired flavor. Make sure the lentils are just heated through in the mixture, because they can get mushy when you reheat the filling for another meal.

PER SERVING Calories: 240; Total fat: 6g; Saturated fat: 2g; Carbs: 40g; Fiber: 11g; Protein: 12g; Sodium: 289mg

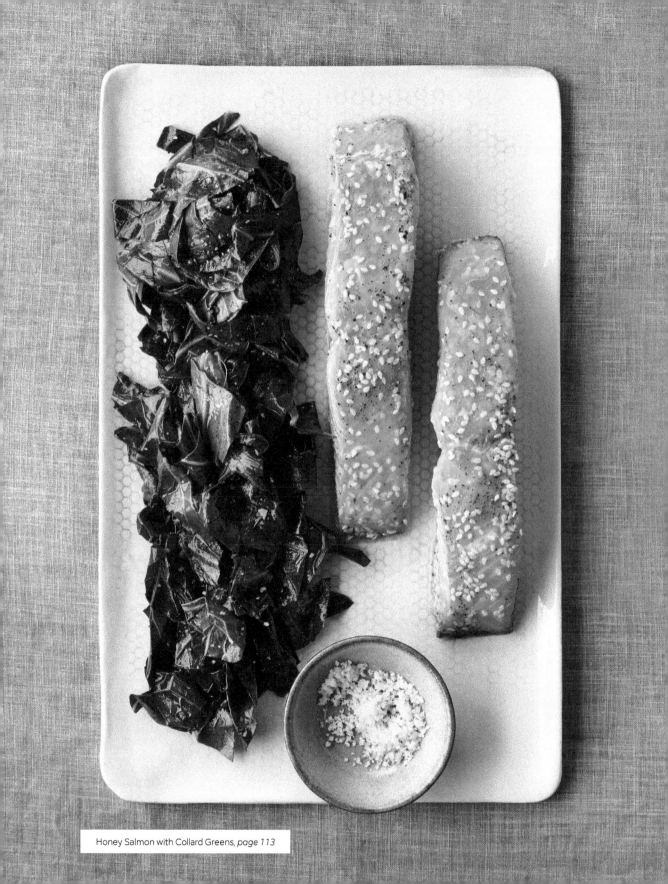

Honey Salmon with Collard Greens, *page 113*

FISH AND SEAFOOD MAINS

QUICK CAJUN SHRIMP AND BROWN RICE

FERTILITY BOOST • INFLAMMATION FIGHTER • WEIGHT MANAGEMENT

ONE-POT

SERVES 4
Prep time: 10 minutes
Cook time: 35 minutes

1 tablespoon olive oil

½ pound (16–10 count) shrimp, peeled and deveined

1 teaspoon Cajun seasoning, divided

1 sweet onion, chopped

2 teaspoons minced garlic

2 cups sodium-free chicken stock

½ cup sodium-free tomato paste

Juice and zest of 1 lime

¾ cup brown rice

Sea salt, for seasoning

Freshly ground black pepper, for seasoning

One cup of brown rice has a glycemic index of 55; however, its glycemic load is only 18. It's a nice addition to a PCOS-focused diet, but in moderation. Brown rice is very high in fiber, so it can regulate blood sugar and hormone levels. It is also a wonderful source of selenium, magnesium, and vitamins B and E.

1. Place a large skillet over medium-high heat and add the olive oil.

2. In a small bowl, toss the shrimp with ¼ teaspoon Cajun seasoning.

3. Sear the shrimp until they are just cooked through, about 5 minutes. Transfer the shrimp to a plate and set aside.

4. Add the onion and garlic to the skillet and sauté until softened, about 5 minutes.

5. Stir in the stock, tomato paste, reserved Cajun seasoning, lime juice, and lime zest.

6. Bring the sauce to a boil and stir in the rice. Then reduce the heat to low, cover, and simmer until the rice is tender, about 20 minutes.

7. Season with salt and pepper.

8. Stir the reserved shrimp into the rice and cook until the shrimp is heated through, about 5 minutes.

PER SERVING Calories: 252; Total fat: 5g; Saturated fat: 1g; Carbs: 32g; Fiber: 4g; Protein: 17g; Sodium: 167mg

SHRIMP PAD THAI

FERTILITY BOOST • WEIGHT MANAGEMENT

ONE-POT

SERVES 4
Prep time: 20 minutes
Cook time: 20 minutes

1 tablespoon olive oil

½ pound (16–20 count) shrimp, peeled and deveined

2 teaspoons grated fresh ginger

1 red bell pepper, julienned

2 cups bean sprouts

2 zucchini, julienned or spiralized

1 cup Tahini Peanut Sauce (page 188)

1 scallion, white and green parts, chopped

2 tablespoons chopped cilantro

2 tablespoons chopped peanuts

Shopping for shrimp requires a bit of homework. You want to ensure that you're purchasing the healthiest, most sustainably caught product. Look for Alaskan pot caught or Canadian giant freshwater prawns farmed in ponds. Shrimp is a spectacular source of vitamin B_{12}, which can help regulate estrogen levels and strengthen the endometrial lining.

1. Place a large skillet over medium-high heat and add the oil.

2. Sauté the shrimp and ginger until they are just cooked through, about 6 minutes.

3. Move the shrimp to the side of the skillet and add the pepper, bean sprouts, and zucchini and sauté until the vegetables are tender crisp, about 6 minutes.

4. Stir in the sauce and toss to coat the shrimp and vegetables. Heat for 5 minutes.

5. Serve topped with scallions, cilantro, and peanuts.

WEIGHT MANAGEMENT TIP: This dish would still be fabulous with just three quarters of the peanut sauce used in the recipe. Cutting the sauce would remove about 50 calories and 4 grams of fat per serving.

PER SERVING Calories: 387; Total fat: 22g; Saturated fat: 5g; Carbs: 21g; Fiber: 6g; Protein: 31g; Sodium: 876mg

FIERY TERIYAKI SHRIMP

FERTILITY BOOST • INFLAMMATION FIGHTER • WEIGHT MANAGEMENT

30-MINUTE

SERVES 4
Prep time: 10 minutes
Cook time: 15 minutes

FOR THE SAUCE

½ cup coconut aminos

¼ cup rice vinegar

3 tablespoons raw honey

1 tablespoon cornstarch

1 tablespoon grated
fresh ginger

1 teaspoon minced garlic

¼ teaspoon chili paste

1 tablespoon olive oil

FOR THE SHRIMP

1 pound (16–20 count)
shrimp, peeled and
deveined

4 cups broccoli florets

Sesame seeds, for garnish

Broccoli is the perfect vegetable for this dish. The top of the florets soak up the sauce and the stems stay slightly firm, adding texture. Broccoli is a fertility superstar. It's packed with vitamin C, iron, and folic acid, which is essential for egg maturation in the ovaries. The iron and folic acid found in broccoli can create a healthy endometrial lining for effective attachment of the zygote, and can help prevent birth defects such as spina bifida.

FOR THE SAUCE

1. In a small bowl, stir together the coconut aminos, vinegar, honey, cornstarch, ginger, garlic, and chili paste.

2. Set aside.

FOR THE SHRIMP

1. Heat the olive oil in a large skillet over medium-high heat.

2. Add the shrimp and sauté for about 6 minutes, until they are just cooked through. Place the shrimp on a plate and set aside.

3. Add the broccoli to the skillet and stir-fry for about 5 minutes, until they're tender crisp.

4. Move the broccoli to the side of the skillet and pour in the sauce. Cook until the sauce thickens, about 2 minutes.

5. Add the shrimp back to the skillet and stir to combine the sauce with the broccoli and shrimp. Serve garnished with the sesame seeds.

INFLAMMATION-FIGHTING TIP: Add sweet bell peppers to perfectly complement this spicy sauce. Bell peppers are a fabulous source of several antioxidants such as carotenoids, lutein, and beta-carotene, which can help reduce inflammation in the body. Whenever possible, use organically grown peppers; their level of antioxidants is higher.

PER SERVING Calories: 280; Total fat: 6g; Saturated fat: 1g; Carbs: 23g; Fiber: 4g; Protein: 31g; Sodium: 1217mg

FIVE-SPICE CALAMARI

FERTILITY BOOST • WEIGHT MANAGEMENT

5-INGREDIENT

SERVES 4
Prep time: 15 minutes,
plus 1 hour
marinating time
Cook time: 10 minutes

1 teaspoon
five-spice powder

1 tablespoon olive oil

4 large squid, cleaned and
split open with tentacles
cut into short lengths

1 red bell pepper, minced

2 tablespoons
chopped cilantro

Zest from 1 lime

Freshly ground black
pepper, for seasoning

Calamari is the Italian word for squid, so don't be surprised if you see tentacles in the package at the supermarket. Fresh squid is obviously the best choice for this dish, but frozen products are still great, thanks to flash-freezing technology on board the ships used to catch the mollusk. Squid is extremely high in protein, copper, iron, and iodine. Iodine is a trace element necessary for proper thyroid function and crucial for manufacturing hormones. Proper thyroid function is necessary for cell division, ovulation, and the development of the fetus.

1. In a medium bowl, stir together the five-spice powder and olive oil.

2. Add the calamari to the marinade and toss.

3. Place the calamari in the refrigerator to marinate for 1 hour.

4. Preheat the oven to broil.

5. Arrange the calamari on a baking sheet in one layer and broil, turning once until just cooked, approximately 10 minutes in total.

6. Place the calamari on a plate and garnish with red pepper, cilantro, lime zest, and black pepper.

INGREDIENT TIP: To save time purchase squid that's been completely cleaned—fresh or frozen. If you decide to clean your own, take care to remove the cuttlebone from the tail portion and the beak.

PER SERVING Calories: 148; Total fat: 5g; Saturated fat: 1g; Carbs: 7g; Fiber: 1g; Protein: 18g; Sodium: 53mg

SEARED SCALLOPS WITH WARM COLESLAW

FERTILITY BOOST • WEIGHT MANAGEMENT

30-MINUTE

SERVES 4
Prep time: 15 minutes
Cook time: 15 minutes

2 tablespoons olive
oil, divided

1 cup Brussels sprouts,
shredded

½ cup shredded
red cabbage

½ cup shredded carrot

1 scallion, white and green
parts, chopped

3 tablespoons apple
cider vinegar

1 tablespoon raw honey

Sea salt, for seasoning

Freshly ground black
pepper, for seasoning

1 pound sea scallops,
cleaned and patted dry

Scallops may not be a common ingredient within your kitchen repertoire, but once you discover how easily they cook, you'll want them in your regular rotation. Scallops are a great source of protein, choline, omega-3 fatty acids, iodine, and vitamin B_{12}, all of which are important for a healthy reproductive system and immune system.

1. Heat 1 tablespoon olive oil in a large skillet over medium-high heat.

2. Add the Brussels sprouts, red cabbage, and carrot and sauté for about 6 minutes, until they're tender crisp.

3. Transfer the vegetables to a bowl and stir in the scallion, vinegar, and honey.

4. Season the slaw with salt and pepper, cover, and set aside.

5. Wipe out the skillet and add the remaining olive oil.

6. Season the scallops with salt and pepper and sear them until golden on both sides, about 4 minutes per side.

7. Serve the scallops with the warm slaw.

VARIATION TIP: Cold coleslaw made with the same ingredients in this recipe, or one of your favorite preparations, would be lovely with these buttery sweet scallops. You can make the slaw ahead and store it in the refrigerator until you're ready to make the scallops.

PER SERVING Calories: 197; Total fat: 8g; Saturated fat: 1g; Carbs: 11g; Fiber: 3g; Protein: 20g; Sodium: 259mg

FISH CURRY WITH KALE

FERTILITY BOOST • WEIGHT MANAGEMENT

**30-MINUTE
ONE-POT**

SERVES 4
Prep time: 10 minutes
Cook time: 20 minutes

1 tablespoon coconut oil

1 sweet onion, chopped

1 teaspoon minced garlic

2 tablespoons
curry powder

1 (15-ounce) can
chopped tomatoes

1 cup coconut milk

½ pound shrimp, peeled
and deveined

½ pound haddock,
cut into 2-inch pieces

2 cups chopped kale

Sea salt, for seasoning

Freshly ground black
pepper, for seasoning

2 tablespoons chopped
fresh cilantro

Fish stews are a quick and flavorful way to access the nutritional benefits of seafood. Even if you aren't a fan of fish, you may find yourself wanting one more bite of the tender fish and creamy sauce. Haddock contains all the essential amino acids and has a lot of protein. It's also rich in lysine, which is crucial for cell growth and calcium absorption—two processes that are needed for a healthy pregnancy.

1. Heat the coconut oil in a large saucepan over medium-high heat.

2. Add the onion and garlic and sauté for about 3 minutes, until softened.

3. Stir in the curry powder.

4. Add the tomatoes and coconut milk and bring to a boil.

5. Stir in the shrimp and fish and reduce the heat to low.

6. Simmer until the seafood is just cooked through, about 10 minutes.

7. Stir in the kale and let the curry sit for 5 minutes to wilt the greens.

8. Season with salt and pepper.

9. Serve topped with cilantro.

SUBSTITUTION TIP: Any firm, fleshy fish works beautifully in this curry. Be sure to purchase the freshest option at your local grocery store or fishmonger. Halibut and salmon are also good choices because they do not flake away when cooked in a sauce or broth.

PER SERVING Calories: 334; Total fat: 19g; Saturated fat: 16g; Carbs: 15g; Fiber: 4g; Protein: 27g; Sodium: 228mg

VEGETABLE BAKED SALMON

FERTILITY BOOST • INFLAMMATION FIGHTER • WEIGHT MANAGEMENT

ONE-PAN

SERVES 4
Prep time: 15 minutes
Cook time: 20 minutes

5 bok choy, quartered and cleaned

2 cups cherry tomatoes

1 sweet onion, thinly sliced

2 teaspoons minced garlic

Juice of 1 lemon

4 (6-ounce) salmon fillets, rinsed and patted dry

Sea salt, for seasoning

Freshly ground black pepper, for seasoning

These parcels filled with tender vegetables and perfectly seasoned fish cooked in its own juices are fun and incredibly easy. There is no stirring involved and you don't even have to supervise the process. Bok choy is a perfect choice of vegetable for this method because as a member of the cabbage family it's sturdy and doesn't overcook. Bok choy is an excellent source of potassium, folate, calcium, and vitamins A, C, and K. The delicate-looking vegetable can reduce the severity of premenstrual syndrome symptoms and fight free radicals in the body.

1. Preheat the oven to 400°F.

2. Tear off three large sheets of foil and place two on a baking sheet, overlapping them in the middle of the pan.

3. In a large bowl, toss together the bok choy, cherry tomatoes, onion, garlic, and lemon juice.

4. Arrange the vegetables in the middle of the foil sheets.

5. Season the fish with salt and pepper and place them on the vegetables in one layer.

6. Lay the third piece of foil on top of the fish and vegetables.

7. Crimp the edges of the foil to make a packet.

8. Cook in the oven until the fish flakes easily with a fork, about 20 minutes.

INFLAMMATION-FIGHTING TIP: Add two carrots cut into small batons to the vegetable mix. This will add a good dose of beta-carotene to the recipe. In the body, beta-carotene is converted into vitamin A, a powerful antioxidant. Carrots are also high in other antioxidants. such as zeaxanthin and lutein.

PER SERVING Calories: 232; Total fat: 6g; Saturated fat: 1g; Carbs: 12g; Fiber: 4g; Protein: 36g; Sodium: 321mg

SPICY CRUSTED HADDOCK WITH CITRUS BASIL SALSA

FERTILITY BOOST • INFLAMMATION FIGHTER • WEIGHT MANAGEMENT

30-MINUTE

SERVES 4
Prep time: 15 minutes
Cook time: 15 minutes

4 (6-ounce) boneless
haddock fillets

½ teaspoon chili powder

Sea salt

Freshly ground
black pepper

1 teaspoon olive oil

1 ruby red grapefruit

1 orange

½ yellow bell pepper, diced

1 scallion, white and
green parts, chopped

2 tablespoons chopped
fresh basil

Haddock is a white-fleshed fish that doesn't have a distinctive "fishy" taste. Its firm texture makes it a perfect candidate for baked fish recipes. If you are concerned about sustainable fishing, look for haddock caught on set longlines or hand lines along the East Coast of the United States. Haddock is a low mercury fish and is very high in vitamin B_{12}, protein, omega-3 fatty acids, zinc, and iron.

1. Preheat the oven to 400°F.

2. Line a baking dish with parchment.

3. Pat the fish dry with paper towels and rub with chili powder.

4. Season the fish lightly with sea salt and pepper.

5. Place the fish in the baking dish in a single layer and drizzle with olive oil.

6. Bake until the fish is light golden brown and flakes easily with a fork, about 12 minutes.

7. While the fish is cooking, cut the skin and pith off the grapefruit and orange, leaving just the flesh. Using a sharp paring knife, section the fruit at the membrane lines. Chop the sections coarsely and transfer them to a bowl with the yellow bell pepper, scallion, and basil.

8. Serve the fish with a generous scoop of salsa.

FERTILITY BOOST: Although the salsa is fresh and colorful, you can add a cup of cannellini beans for a fertility-friendly dish. It will only increase the calorie count by about 25 per serving. Cannellini beans are a great source of many fertility-boosting nutrients such as folate and choline.

PER SERVING Calories: 202; Total fat: 3g; Saturated fat: 0g; Carbs: 10g; Fiber: 2g; Protein: 33g; Sodium: 205mg

SUN-DRIED TOMATO BAKED COD

FERTILITY BOOST • INFLAMMATION FIGHTER • WEIGHT MANAGEMENT

30-MINUTE
ONE-POT

SERVES 4
Prep time: 10 minutes
Cook time: 20 minutes

2 tablespoons olive oil

1 sweet onion, sliced

2 teaspoons minced garlic

1 (15-ounce) can
sodium-free diced
tomatoes

½ cup sun-dried
tomatoes, chopped

2 teaspoons dried basil

Pinch red pepper flakes

Sea salt, for seasoning

Freshly ground black
pepper, for seasoning

4 (6-ounce) cod fillets

Cod contains many of the nutrients that make fish a wonderful choice for a healthy diet. This includes protein, vitamins B_6 and B_{12}, along with omega-3 fatty acids, and selenium. Cod can help fight inflammation and boost fertility. The sun-dried tomatoes add protein, zinc, and calcium, giving the dish a double dose of protein. This can help produce better egg quality and implantation of the fertilized egg.

1. Preheat the oven to 400°F.

2. Heat the olive oil in an oven-safe large skillet over medium-high heat.

3. Add the onion and garlic and sauté for about 3 minutes until softened.

4. Stir in tomatoes, sun-dried tomatoes, basil, and red pepper flakes.

5. Season with salt and pepper.

6. Push the sauce to the edges of the skillet and add the cod in one layer.

7. Spoon the sauce over the fish and bake until the fish is opaque and flakes easily, about 15 to 17 minutes.

8. Remove the skillet from the oven and serve.

FERTILITY BOOST TIP: Halibut would work well in this dish. It's an excellent source of selenium, about 60 milligrams per serving which is close to 90 percent of the daily recommended amount for good reproductive health. Selenium is a powerful antioxidant and can help protect the embryo from chromosomal damage.

PER SERVING Calories: 239; Total fat: 9g; Saturated fat: 1g; Carbs: 11g; Fiber: 4g; Protein: 33g; Sodium: 324mg

TROUT WITH TOMATO-PEPPER RELISH

INFLAMMATION FIGHTER • WEIGHT MANAGEMENT

30-MINUTE

SERVES 4
Prep time: 15 minutes
Cook time: 15 minutes

FOR THE RELISH

1 cup tomatoes, chopped

1 cup roasted red bell pepper, chopped

½ jalapeño pepper, minced

2 tablespoons chopped fresh cilantro

FOR THE FISH

4 (6-ounce) trout fillets

1 teaspoon ground cumin

Sea salt

Freshly ground black pepper

Olive oil, for greasing the baking dish

Relish is usually a cooked condiment. But the chopped red bell pepper used in this recipe creates a smoother texture, as opposed to salsa, so relish seemed like an appropriate description. The bright color and heat in the relish indicates the presence of beta-carotene (red bell peppers) and capsaicin (jalapeños), both potent anti-inflammatories.

FOR THE RELISH

1. In a small bowl, stir together the tomatoes, red bell pepper, jalapeño pepper, and cilantro.

2. Set aside.

FOR THE FISH

1. Preheat the oven to 400°F.

2. Season the fish on both sides with cumin, salt, and pepper.

3. Place the fish on a lightly oiled baking sheet and roast in the oven until the flesh is fork tender, about 15 minutes.

4. Serve the fish with the tomato-pepper relish.

FERTILITY BOOST TIP: Salmon is also another excellent choice to serve with this fresh salsa and it cooks in the same time. Salmon is high in coenzyme Q_{10}, which is an important antioxidant for fertility. CoQ_{10} can protect DNA from damage and increase ova (egg) health.

PER SERVING Calories: 241; Total fat: 11g; Saturated fat: 3g; Carbs: 5g; Fiber: 1g; Protein: 32g; Sodium: 138mg

PAN-SEARED TROUT WITH CREAMY LEMON SAUCE

FERTILITY BOOST • INFLAMMATION FIGHTER • WEIGHT MANAGEMENT

30-MINUTE

SERVES 4
Prep time: 10 minutes
Cook time: 20 minutes

1 tablespoon olive oil

4 (6-ounce) trout fillets

¼ cup freshly squeezed lemon juice

1 tablespoon cornstarch

1 tablespoon lemon zest

1 tablespoon raw honey

1 teaspoon fresh thyme, chopped

½ cup low-fat plain Greek yogurt

2 tablespoons scallion greens, chopped

Anyone who has grown up near fresh water lakes has probably enjoyed a shore lunch of freshly caught trout. This sweet-tasting fish is low in mercury. In grocery stores trout is sometimes displayed in tanks so you don't have to break out your fishing rod. The fish is high in protein and omega-3 fatty acids, which supports fertility by helping produce good-quality eggs. It also fights inflammation.

1. Preheat the oven to 400°F.

2. Heat the olive oil in a large oven-safe skillet over medium-high heat.

3. Pan sear the trout on both sides for about 6 minutes and place the skillet in the oven until the fish is just cooked through, about 15 to 18 minutes.

4. Make the sauce while the fish is baking.

5. In a small saucepan over medium-high heat, whisk together the lemon juice, cornstarch, zest, honey, and thyme for about 3 minutes, until the mixture thickens.

6. Remove the sauce from the heat and whisk in the yogurt.

7. Serve the fish with the sauce and topped with scallions.

FERTILITY BOOST TIP: Serve this light and delicious main course with a generous scoop of fresh green peas. Peas are high in zinc, which is crucial for boosting fertility. Estrogen and progesterone levels can be negatively affected by a zinc deficiency.

PER SERVING Calories: 295; Total fat: 12g; Saturated fat: 1g; Carbs: 9g; Fiber: 1g; Protein: 35g; Sodium: 26mg

LIME-POACHED HALIBUT

INFLAMMATION FIGHTER • WEIGHT MANAGEMENT

BULK COOK

SERVES 4
Prep time: 15 minutes
Cook time: 1 hour

6 cups water

Juice and zest of 2 limes

1 sweet onion, sliced

3 celery stalks, with the greens, coarsely chopped

1 carrot, coarsely chopped

2 garlic cloves, crushed

2 dill sprigs

2 thyme sprigs

1 bay leaf

¼ teaspoon black peppercorns

¼ teaspoon sea salt

4 (6-ounce) halibut fillets or 1 side of fish

Poaching has a reputation as a dry preparation for fish. This usually occurs if you leave the fillet in the liquid for too long, creating a tough texture. However, when done properly, poached fish is delectable and incredibly versatile. When making the court bouillon—the poaching liquid—take the time to taste it because the flavors in the broth will infuse the fish.

1. Add the water, lime juice, lime zest, onion, celery, carrot, garlic, dill, thyme, bay leaf, peppercorns, and salt to a large pot over medium-high heat.

2. Bring the liquid to boil and then reduce the heat to low and simmer for 45 minutes.

3. Strain the poaching liquid through a sieve into a large skillet on low heat.

4. Place the fish in the poaching liquid and cover.

5. Simmer the halibut for 10 minutes, until the fish is opaque and just cooked through.

6. Remove the fish carefully and serve.

BULK COOKING TIP: Delicately poached fish is a must-have ingredient to have on hand for salads, wraps, and other recipes. You can store it for 3 days in a sealed plastic bag in the refrigerator. If you freeze the fish, only use it for salad fillings or fish cakes, because the texture tends to get mushy when it's thawed.

PER SERVING Calories: 228; Total fat: 4g; Saturated fat: 0g; Carbs: 2g; Fiber: 0g; Protein: 46g; Sodium: 248mg

HONEY SALMON WITH COLLARD GREENS

INFLAMMATION FIGHTER • WEIGHT MANAGEMENT

30-MINUTE

SERVES 4
Prep time: 10 minutes
Cook time: 20 minutes

4 (6-ounce) salmon fillets, patted dry

Sea salt, for seasoning

Freshly ground black pepper, for seasoning

2 tablespoons raw honey

2 tablespoons sesame seeds

1 tablespoon olive oil

4 cups chopped collard greens

Honey and sesame are a classic pairing, found in centuries-old recipes, often created for wellness and fertility. The mixture of sesame and honey is an excellent source of essential amino acids, omega-3 fatty acids, calcium, iron, manganese, and magnesium. Together, honey and sesame can reduce stress, increase energy, strengthen bones, and stimulate mental activity.

1. Preheat the oven to 400°F.

2. Lightly season the fish with salt and pepper.

3. Line a baking dish with parchment and place the fish in the dish.

4. Spread the honey on top of the fillets and sprinkle with sesame seeds.

5. Bake the salmon for 15 to 17 minutes, until it is just cooked through.

6. While the fish is baking, add the olive oil to a large skillet over medium-high heat.

7. Add the collard greens and sauté for about 10 minutes, until tender and bright green.

8. Season the greens with salt and pepper.

9. Serve the fish on a generous scoop of sautéed greens.

INGREDIENT TIP: Collard greens are available in most grocery stores in the refrigerator case of the produce section. Unrefrigerated collard greens can be bitter and wilted. Look for properly chilled greens with firm, deep green leaves with no browning. The most mild and tender greens will have small and sturdy leaves.

PER SERVING Calories: 300; Total fat: 18g; Saturated fat: 3g; Carbs: 11g; Fiber: 2g; Protein: 24g; Sodium: 123mg

DILL SALMON BURGERS

FERTILITY BOOST • INFLAMMATION FIGHTER • WEIGHT MANAGEMENT

BULK COOK

SERVES 4
Prep time: 10 minutes, plus 30 minutes chilling time; Cook time: 14 minutes

½ pound cooked boneless salmon fillet

¾ cup almond flour

1 scallion, white and green parts, chopped

¼ cup shredded carrot

1 egg, beaten

Juice and zest of 1 lemon

1 tablespoon dill, chopped

Sea salt, for seasoning

Freshly ground black pepper, for seasoning

1 tablespoon olive oil

4 sprouted grain buns

Favorite toppings

Salmon is a healthy fatty fish known for its omega-3 fatty acids, which can regulate hormones and stimulate blood flow to the ovaries, fallopian tubes, and uterus. Salmon has low amounts of mercury, so it can be enjoyed once a week on a PCOS diet. Dill has a marvelous anise flavor that works well with the salmon, sweet carrot, and the citrus in this recipe. Dill contains the essential oil eugenol, which can reduce blood sugar.

1. In a large bowl, mix together the salmon, almond flour, scallion, carrot, egg, lemon juice, lemon zest, and dill until the mixture holds together when pressed.

2. Season the salmon mixture with salt and pepper.

3. Place the salmon mixture in the refrigerator and chill for 30 minutes.

4. Divide the salmon mixture into four portions and press them into patties, about ½-inch thick.

5. Heat the olive oil in a large skillet over medium-high heat.

6. Cook the salmon patties for about 7 minutes on each side. Only turn them once.

7. Serve on buns with your favorite toppings.

BULK COOKING TIP: Cook these burgers before freezing. When you are ready to store them, lay the patties flat on a baking tray and place in the freezer. Once frozen transfer them to a plastic freezer bag. If you don't have room in your freezer for a baking tray, separate the burgers with squares of parchment inside a plastic freezer bag so you can take them out individually.

PER SERVING Calories: 254; Total fat: 12g; Saturated fat: 2g; Carbs: 20g; Fiber: 4g; Protein: 17g; Sodium: 236mg

SEAFOOD STEW

FERTILITY BOOST • INFLAMMATION FIGHTER • WEIGHT MANAGEMENT

ONE-POT

SERVES 4
Prep time: 15 minutes
Cook time: 40 minutes

1 tablespoon olive oil

1 sweet onion, chopped

1 tablespoon
minced garlic

2 parsnips, diced

3 cups sodium-free
vegetable or fish
stock, divided

1 (15-ounce) can
sodium-free diced
tomatoes

½ pound firm white flesh
fish, cut into 1-inch cubes

¼ pound shrimp, peeled
and deveined

20 bay scallops

2 tablespoons cornstarch
to thicken

Sea salt, for seasoning

Freshly ground black
pepper, for seasoning

Stew usually requires hours to properly tenderize meats or poultry. This quick seafood version is a nice change because it's on the table in less than 1 hour. You can certainly use whatever vegetables you have in the refrigerator, but try to keep the parsnips in the recipe if possible. They add a glorious earthy flavor and tons of fiber. This can help stabilize blood sugar and keep you feeling full longer.

1. Heat the olive oil in a medium stockpot over medium-high heat.

2. Add the onion and garlic and sauté for about 4 minutes, until softened.

3. Stir in the parsnip and sauté for 1 minute.

4. Stir in 2½ cups stock and diced tomatoes.

5. Bring the stew to a boil, reduce the heat to low and simmer for 20 minutes, until the vegetables are tender.

6. Stir in the fish, shrimp, and scallops and simmer for about 10 minutes, until the seafood is just cooked through.

7. In a small bowl, stir together the remaining stock and cornstarch.

8. Add the cornstarch mixture to the stew and stir until the stew thickens, about 2 minutes.

9. Season the stew with salt and pepper.

INFLAMMATION-FIGHTING TIP: Herbs have amazing medicinal properties, so adding them to recipes brings more than just wonderful flavor. Add 2 tablespoons of chopped basil to this soup to access the powerful anti-inflammatory and antibacterial properties of these herbs.

PER SERVING Calories: 270; Total fat: 6g; Saturated fat: 1g; Carbs: 26g; Fiber: 7g; Protein: 28g; Sodium: 353mg

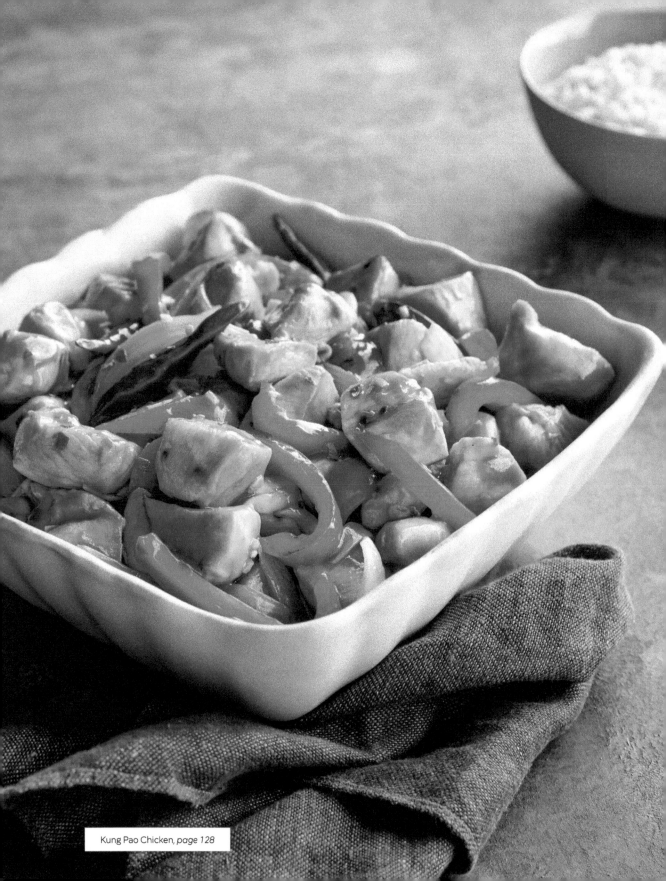

Kung Pao Chicken, *page 128*

CHICKEN AND TURKEY MAINS

CHICKEN-ALMOND MEATLOAF

FERTILITY BOOST • INFLAMMATION FIGHTER • WEIGHT MANAGEMENT

BULK COOK

SERVES 4
Prep time: 10 minutes
Cook time: 1 hour

1 pound lean
ground chicken

½ cup almond flour

½ cup grated carrot

1 scallion, white and
green parts, chopped

½ red bell pepper,
finely chopped

2 teaspoons minced garlic

1 teaspoon grated
fresh ginger

1 egg

Sea salt, for seasoning

Freshly ground black
pepper, for seasoning

Meatloaf is the epitome of comfort food; It's tasty and easy to prepare. Ground chicken is lighter than beef or pork and combines well with the golden almonds and generous amounts of fresh ginger and garlic. Ground chicken breast is also lean and high in protein. You can purchase ground chicken with thigh meat for a slightly juicier texture.

1. Preheat the oven to 350°F.

2. Line an 8-by-4-inch loaf pan with parchment paper and set aside.

3. In a large bowl, mix together the chicken, almond flour, carrot, scallion, red bell pepper, garlic, ginger, and egg until well combined.

4. Season the mixture with salt and pepper.

5. Pack the meatloaf into the loaf pan and bake until the meatloaf is cooked through and golden on top, about 1 hour.

6. Remove the meatloaf from the oven and let stand for 10 minutes.

7. Drain off any visible grease before serving.

BULK COOKING TIP: You can cook this juicy meatloaf from frozen or after thawing in the refrigerator overnight. If you're cooking it after thawing, follow the timing in the recipe. If you're popping the dish directly from the freezer into the oven, cook between 1½ and 2 hours or until the internal temperature reaches 165°F.

PER SERVING Calories: 202; Total fat: 9g; Saturated fat: 3g; Carbs: 4g; Fiber: 1g; Protein: 27g; Sodium: 211mg

CHICKEN-CAULIFLOWER CASSEROLE

FERTILITY BOOST • WEIGHT MANAGEMENT

BULK COOK

SERVES 4
Prep time: 10 minutes
Cook time: 40 minutes

3 cups chopped cooked
chicken breasts

2 cups cooked quinoa

3 cups cauliflower florets,
blanched

1 tablespoon olive oil

1 sweet onion, chopped

2 teaspoons minced garlic

2 tablespoons cornstarch

1 cup sodium-free
chicken stock

½ cup coconut milk

Sea salt, for seasoning

Freshly ground black
pepper, for seasoning

You may be more familiar with the casserole that inspired this dish—chicken divine. The cauliflower replaces broccoli and there is no cheese in this version. The chicken breast still takes center stage because it is a great source of protein, about 21 grams per 100 grams of chicken breast. Chicken is also high in vitamin B_6, a crucial micronutrient for hormone balance. It's particularly good at reducing excessive androgen and testosterone in the blood.

1. Preheat the oven to 350°F.

2. In a large bowl, toss together the chicken, quinoa, and cauliflower and set aside.

3. Heat the olive oil in a small saucepan over medium-high heat.

4. Add the onion and garlic and sauté until softened, about 3 minutes.

5. Whisk in the cornstarch and cook 1 minute.

6. Whisk in the chicken stock and coconut milk to form a thick sauce, about 4 to 5 minutes.

7. Season the sauce with salt and pepper.

8. Add the sauce to the large bowl and stir to coat the chicken, quinoa, and cauliflower.

CONTINUED

9. Transfer the mixture to a large casserole dish.

10. Bake the casserole for 20 to 30 minutes, until warmed through.

BULK COOKING TIP: You can freeze casseroles that are cooked or uncooked. Depending on your preference, just thaw the dish in the refrigerator overnight before popping it into the oven. This recipe can be doubled or tripled with no changes to the spicing or quantities.

PER SERVING Calories: 435; Total fat: 18g; Saturated fat: 8g; Carbs: 32g; Fiber: 7g; Protein: 32g; Sodium: 150mg

CHICKEN CHILI FAJITAS

FERTILITY BOOST • INFLAMMATION FIGHTER

ONE-POT

SERVES 4
Prep time: 15 minutes
Cook time: 20 minutes

1 tablespoon olive oil

4 (5-ounce) boneless skinless chicken breasts, cut into strips

1 red onion, thinly sliced

1 red bell pepper, cut into thin strips

1 yellow bell pepper, cut into thin strips

1 green bell pepper, cut into thin strips

2 teaspoons minced garlic

1 tablespoon Tex-Mex seasoning

4 sprouted grain tortillas

Traditionally, fajitas come served on an insanely hot sizzling cast iron. This simple preparation considerably reduces the risk of burn. Chicken breast is thinly sliced and sautéed until lightly browned and juicy. Chicken is very rich in B vitamins, potassium, amino acids, and potassium. The B vitamins help balance hormones and are crucial for zinc absorption.

1. Heat the olive oil in a large skillet over medium-high heat.

2. Sauté the chicken strips for about 10 minutes, until they're just cooked through. Remove the chicken with a slotted spoon to small bowl.

3. Put the skillet back on heat and add onion, peppers, and garlic and sauté for about 6 minutes, until they're lightly caramelized and nearly tender.

4. Stir in seasoning and reserved chicken strips and juices.

5. Sauté for 5 minutes more.

6. Spoon the filling onto the tortillas and roll them up.

INFLAMMATION-FIGHTING TIP: Serve the fajitas with a couple tablespoons of chopped avocado to add a cool, creamy element to the dish. Avocado is high in omega-3 fatty acids, about 190 milligrams per 100 grams of fruit, as well as inflammation-busting vitamin E.

PER SERVING Calories: 362; Total fat: 9g; Saturated fat: 1g; Carbs: 34g; Fiber: 7g; Protein: 36g; Sodium: 221mg

SALSA VERDE CHICKEN

INFLAMMATION FIGHTER • WEIGHT MANAGEMENT

ONE-POT

SERVES 4
Prep time: 10 minutes
Cook time: 45 minutes

1 pound boneless, skinless chicken thighs

Sea salt, for seasoning

Freshly ground black pepper, for seasoning

1 tablespoon olive oil

2 cups chopped fresh spinach

2 cups prepared salsa verde

2 tablespoons chopped fresh cilantro

Lime, cut into wedges, for garnish

Salsa verde is made from the nightshade vegetable called a tomatillo. It's closely related to a gooseberry, even though in appearance it looks like a green tomato covered in a husk. Tomatillos are very rich in dietary fiber, potassium, magnesium, and manganese, and high in vitamins A, C, and K. This small green vegetable can help you feel full longer, boost your immune system, and reduce your risk of heart disease and diabetes.

1. Preheat the oven to 400°F.

2. Season the chicken with salt and pepper.

3. Heat the olive oil in an oven-safe large skillet over medium-high heat.

4. Brown the chicken on both sides for about 4 minutes each.

5. Remove the skillet from the heat and push the chicken to the side of the skillet.

6. Spread the spinach in the bottom of the skillet and place the chicken on top.

7. Pour the salsa verde over the chicken.

8. Bake until the chicken is cooked through, about 35 minutes.

9. Remove the chicken from the oven.

10. Serve topped with cilantro and lime wedges.

FERTILITY BOOST TIP: Spread 1 cup of black beans over the spinach before placing the chicken on top. It will increase the fiber content, which helps regulate blood sugar. Black beans are very high in phytoestrogen, as well, so this ingredient supports the maturation of healthy eggs.

PER SERVING Calories: 194; Total fat: 8g; Saturated fat: 2g; Carbs: 6g; Fiber: 1g; Protein: 24g; Sodium: 24mg

PESTO CHICKEN EN PAPILLOTE

FERTILITY BOOST • INFLAMMATION FIGHTER • WEIGHT MANAGEMENT

ONE-PAN

SERVES 4
Prep time: 10 minutes
Cook time: 30 minutes

4 (4-ounce) skinless,
boneless chicken breast,
cut in half horizontally

4 cups packed
chopped kale

2 cups shiitake
mushrooms, sliced

1 red bell pepper, diced

½ cup sun-dried
tomato pesto

2 tablespoons chopped
fresh basil

½ cup sodium-free
chicken stock

Freshly ground black
pepper, for seasoning

In the strictest sense, *en papillote* is French for cooking in a paper parcel, so the foil in this preparation is a bit of a stretch. But it's easier to fold and crimp foil than paper into a sealed packet. Cooking in foil ensures that every drop of juice stays in the poultry and greens; no flavor escapes at all. Be careful when opening the packet because there will be a burst of steam that can burn your hands.

1. Preheat the oven to 400°F.

2. Tear off four large pieces of foil and lay them on a clean work surface.

3. Arrange the chicken breasts on the foil pieces so the two halves form a single layer.

4. Top each chicken breast with one-fourth of the kale, mushrooms, red bell pepper, sun-dried tomato pesto, and basil.

5. Fold the edges of the foil up and add 2 tablespoons chicken stock to the packets. Season each packet with pepper.

6. Fold the edges over the ingredients to completely enclose them and crimp the edges.

7. Transfer the packets to a baking sheet and bake until the chicken is cooked through, about 30 minutes.

FERTILITY BOOST TIP: Kale is rich in iron, so add a couple extra cups to increase your intake of the mineral. You need to consume about 27 milligrams iron per day for healthy fertility. Iron deficiency can cause lack of ovulation and create poor egg health.

PER SERVING Calories: 205; Total fat: 5g; Saturated fat: 2g; Carbs: 11g; Fiber: 2g; Protein: 29g; Sodium: 222mg

LEMON CHICKEN WITH OLIVES

FERTILITY BOOST • INFLAMMATION FIGHTER • WEIGHT MANAGEMENT

30-MINUTE

SERVES 4
Prep time: 15 minutes
Cook time: 15 minutes

4 (5-ounce) skinless, boneless chicken breast, pounded flat to ½-inch thickness

1 egg

¼ cup coconut milk

1 cup almond flour

1 tablespoon olive oil

1 cup sodium-free chicken stock

Juice and zest from 2 lemons

2 tablespoons raw honey

1 tablespoon cornstarch

¼ cup Kalamata olives, sliced

1 scallion, white and green parts, sliced

Lemon and olives are a traditional pairing in Greek and Mediterranean food. Citrus trees can be found in all regions of Greece, so their flavor is very common in authentic recipes, while olive groves are a farming industry staple that spans thousands of years in the country. In this recipe, the tart lemon sauce and chopped black olives are served with juicy lightly browned breaded chicken strips. Delicious.

1. Preheat the oven to 400°F.

2. Line a baking sheet with parchment and set aside.

3. Whisk together the egg and coconut milk in a small bowl.

4. Place the almond flour in a bowl next to the egg mixture.

5. Dredge the chicken in the egg mixture and then coat in the almond flour.

6. Place the chicken on the baking sheet and brush lightly with olive oil.

7. Bake for about 15 minutes, until cooked through.

8. While the chicken is cooking, place a small saucepan over medium heat and add the chicken stock, lemon juice, lemon zest, honey, and cornstarch.

9. Whisk the sauce for about 5 minutes, until it's thick and creamy.

10. Stir in the olives.

11. Serve the breaded chicken with the lemon sauce and topped with the scallion.

FERTILITY BOOST TIP: Try to have at least one serving of citrus fruit per day such as the lemons in this luscious sauce. Citrus fruit is rich in vitamin C, folate, calcium, and potassium, which can help regulate ovulation and fight inflammation.

PER SERVING Calories: 348; Total fat: 17g; Saturated fat: 6g; Carbs: 13g; Fiber: 2g; Protein: 35g; Sodium: 143mg

CREAMY CHICKEN PAPRIKASH

FERTILITY BOOST • WEIGHT MANAGEMENT

ONE-POT

SERVES 4
Prep time: 10 minutes
Cook time: 35 minutes

1 tablespoon olive oil

1 pound skinless, boneless chicken thighs, cut into 1-inch pieces

1 sweet onion, chopped

1 red bell pepper, chopped

2 tablespoons sweet paprika

¼ teaspoon sea salt

¼ teaspoon freshly ground black pepper

1 (15-ounce) can sodium-free diced tomatoes, undrained

1 cup sodium-free chicken stock

½ cup spinach

½ cup low-fat plain Greek yogurt

1 tablespoon cornstarch

¼ cup chopped fresh parsley

The parsley and spinach bring a vibrant note of bright green in this pretty red sauce. The added color is well worth it; these ingredients can alleviate painful PMS symptoms. Spinach is high in zinc, vitamin B_6, and vitamin C, which can reduce the severity of hormone-related cramps. Parsley contains a cramp-relieving compound called apiole, which doubles the positive impact of spinach.

1. Heat the olive oil in a large skillet on medium-high heat.

2. Add the chicken and sauté until it's browned on both sides, about 10 minutes in total.

3. Add the onion, red bell pepper, paprika, salt, and pepper and sauté for 3 minutes.

4. Stir in the tomatoes and chicken stock and bring the liquid to a boil.

5. Reduce the heat to low and simmer for about 20 minutes, until the chicken is tender.

6. Stir in the spinach in the last 5 minutes.

7. Stir the cornstarch into the yogurt and add the mixture to the sauce, stirring for about 2 minutes, until it thickens.

8. Serve topped with parsley.

FERTILITY BOOST TIP: Turkey is smart choice for this dish if you want to change the traditional preparation. The white meat is high in vitamin B_6, a crucial fertility vitamin. Vitamin B_6 can increase menstruation's luteal phase and increase the health of the eggs.

PER SERVING Calories: 244; Total fat: 8g; Saturated fat: 2g; Carbs: 13g; Fiber: 3g; Protein: 30g; Sodium: 215mg

RICH ROASTED RED PEPPER CHICKEN

FERTILITY BOOST • INFLAMMATION FIGHTER • WEIGHT MANAGEMENT

ONE-POT

SERVES 4
Prep time: 10 minutes
Cook time: 35 minutes

1 tablespoon olive oil

1 pound boneless skinless chicken breast, cut into strips

1 sweet onion, chopped

1 tablespoon minced garlic

2 cups canned or jarred roasted red peppers, finely chopped

1 cup sodium-free chicken stock

½ cup sun-dried tomatoes, chopped

½ cup coconut cream

⅛ teaspoon red pepper flakes

Sea salt, for seasoning

Freshly ground black pepper, for seasoning

¼ cup chopped fresh basil

This sauce is a culinary revelation. You may find yourself scraping the plate with a spoon to get every last drop of the sauce. Sun-dried tomatoes, coconut cream, garlic, rich smoky red pepper, and a touch of heat blend really well, for a sublime finish. This sauce could be used for shrimp, flaky white fish, pork, or chicken. Oven roast your own tomatoes in a 250°F oven for about 3 hours if you have the time.

1. Heat the olive oil in a large skillet over medium-high heat.

2. Add the chicken and sauté for about 15 minutes, until it is lightly browned and just cooked through.

3. Remove the chicken to a plate with a slotted spoon.

4. Add the onion and garlic and sauté for about 3 minutes, until softened.

5. Stir in the roasted red peppers, chicken stock, sun-dried tomatoes, coconut cream, and red pepper flakes.

6. Bring the sauce to a boil and then reduce the heat to low and simmer for about 10 minutes, until the sauce reduces by one quarter.

7. Season the sauce with salt and pepper and return the chicken to the sauce with any accumulated juice.

8. Simmer for 4 minutes more.

9. Serve topped with basil.

INFLAMMATION-FIGHTING TIP: Stir in a cup of halved cherry tomatoes along with the roasted red tomatoes to boost the antioxidant content of this dish. Tomatoes contain lycopene. The antioxidant boosts the available amount of this phytochemical by about 35 percent.

PER SERVING Calories: 316; Total fat: 15g; Saturated fat: 7g; Carbs: 14g; Fiber: 3g; Protein: 33g; Sodium: 310mg

KUNG PAO CHICKEN

INFLAMMATION FIGHTER • WEIGHT MANAGEMENT

**30-MINUTE
ONE-POT**

SERVES 4

Prep time: 10 minutes
Cook time: 20 minutes

1 tablespoon sesame oil

3 (5-ounce) boneless
skinless chicken breasts,
cut into 1-inch chunks

1 sweet onion, cut
into eighths

3 red bell peppers, cut
into strips

1 tablespoon
minced garlic

1 cup sodium-free
chicken stock divided

3 tablespoons
coconut aminos

3 tablespoons chili paste

1 tablespoon molasses

¼ teaspoon red
pepper flakes

1 tablespoon cornstarch

This is a variation on an authentic Kung Pao chicken recipe. It's missing the fried peanuts and Shaoxing Chinese cooking wine, but you won't notice. The pepper strips in this version add bulk and important antioxidants and nutrients to the meal. If you happen to have a good Asian market in your neighborhood, substitute 6 whole dried Chinese chili peppers for the chili paste.

1. Heat the sesame oil in a large skillet over medium-high heat.

2. Add the chicken and sauté until for about 12 minutes, until it's cooked through and lightly browned.

3. Remove the chicken to a plate with a slotted spoon.

4. Add the onion, peppers, and garlic and sauté for about 6 minutes, until the vegetables are lightly caramelized.

5. In a small bowl, whisk together ¾ cup chicken stock, coconut aminos, chili paste, molasses, and red pepper flakes.

6. Pour the sauce into the skillet and add the reserved chicken and any accumulated juice from the plate.

7. In the same small bowl stir together the remaining chicken stock and the cornstarch.

8. Bring the sauce to a boil and then pour in the cornstarch mixture.

9. Stir for about 2 minutes, until the sauce is thick.

FERTILITY BOOST TIP: Choline is an essential nutrient for fetal development, so including foods rich in this nutrient to your diet is important. Cauliflower is very high in choline, so try adding 1 cup of small florets to this dish.

PER SERVING Calories: 253; Total fat: 8g; Saturated fat: 1g; Carbs: 18g; Fiber: 2g; Protein: 26g; Sodium: 716mg

GARLIC CHICKEN THIGHS WITH LENTILS AND ASPARAGUS

FERTILITY BOOST · INFLAMMATION FIGHTER · WEIGHT MANAGEMENT

5-INGREDIENT

SERVES 4
Prep time: 10 minutes
Cook time: 35 minutes

2 tablespoons olive oil

4 (5-ounce) bone-in skinless chicken thighs

1 teaspoon garlic powder

Sea salt, for seasoning

Freshly ground black pepper, for seasoning

2 cups canned sodium-free lentils

12-15 asparagus spears, cut into 1-inch pieces

2 cups cherry tomatoes, halved

Asparagus is an often-underutilized vegetable. That is likely due to its limited seasonal availability and its sensitivity to heat—if it isn't cooked correctly the green stalks can quickly turn gray and limp. But don't let that discourage you. Asparagus is an exceptionally good source of vitamin K, folate, and more than 100 inflammation-busting phytonutrients. Folate is important for preventing birth defects. The other compounds in asparagus such as 2"-dihydroxynicotianamine are linked to better regulation of blood sugar.

1. Preheat the oven to 400°F.

2. Heat the olive oil in a large ovenproof skillet over medium-high heat

3. Season the chicken thighs lightly with garlic powder, salt, and pepper, and pan sear skin side down until crispy and golden, about 10 minutes.

4. Turn the chicken over and place the skillet in the oven, roasting until the chicken is cooked through, 20 to 25 minutes.

CONTINUED

5. Remove the skillet from the oven and transfer the chicken thighs to a plate.

6. Place the skillet back over medium-high heat, taking care because it is hot, and add the lentils, asparagus, and tomatoes.

7. Stir until the legumes are heated through and the asparagus is tender, about 5 minutes.

8. Serve the chicken over the lentil mixture.

VARIATION TIP: Leave the skin on when cooking to create a delicious moist chicken thigh. Then remove the skin before serving to reduce the saturated fat and total fat in this dish.

PER SERVING Calories: 340; Total fat: 17g; Saturated fat: 4g; Carbs: 26g; Fiber: 10g; Protein: 28g; Sodium: 77mg

FOOLPROOF ROASTED CHICKEN

FERTILITY BOOST · INFLAMMATION FIGHTER · WEIGHT MANAGEMENT

5-INGREDIENT
BULK COOK

SERVES 4
Prep time: 10 minutes
Cook time: 30 minutes

1 teaspoon garlic powder

½ teaspoon dried oregano

½ teaspoon dried thyme

Pinch sea salt

Pinch freshly ground
black pepper

1 tablespoon olive oil

4 (5-ounce) boneless
skinless chicken breasts

Roasted chicken is one of the most versatile dishes. It works as the centerpiece of a lovely dinner but also as leftovers for salads, sandwiches, and soups. The best strategy when creating this simple recipe is to double it and use the leftovers for other meals and snacks. To properly store the chicken, first chill the extra breast meat in the refrigerator, then place it in sealed plastic bags. Keep the chicken in the refrigerator for up to 4 days or in the freezer for 1 month.

1. Preheat the oven to 375°F.

2. Stir together garlic powder, oregano, thyme, salt, and pepper in a small bowl.

3. Rub the chicken breasts all over with the spice mixture.

4. Heat the olive oil in a large ovenproof skillet over medium-high heat.

5. Pan sear the chicken breasts until golden, turning once, about 10 minutes in total.

6. Place the skillet in the oven and roast until the chicken is cooked through, 20 to 25 minutes.

INFLAMMATION-FIGHTING TIP: Mix in ¼ teaspoon ground turmeric with the spices to add an active compound called curcumin to the dish. Curcumin is a powerful anti-inflammatory that can block the production of inflammation-causing enzymes in the body.

PER SERVING Calories: 213; Total fat: 6g; Saturated fat: 1g; Carbs: 1g; Fiber: 0g; Protein: 35g; Sodium: 171mg

MUSHROOM CHICKEN THIGHS

FERTILITY BOOST • INFLAMMATION FIGHTER • WEIGHT MANAGEMENT

5-INGREDIENT

SERVES 4
Prep time: 10 minutes
Cook time: 45 minutes

3 tablespoons olive oil, divided

4 cups sliced wild mushrooms

2 teaspoons minced garlic

1 teaspoon fresh thyme, chopped

4 (6-ounce) bone-in chicken thighs

Sea salt, for seasoning

Freshly ground black pepper, for seasoning

Caramelized mushrooms are a culinary triumph and adding garlic and thyme only enhances their richness of flavor. Mushrooms are a fabulous source of vitamin D, which when added to thyme is a powerful anti-inflammatory combination. Thyme is high in volatile oils, flavonoids, manganese, vitamin A, and vitamin C, all of which fight inflammation and reduce free radicals in the body.

1. Preheat the oven to 425°F.

2. Heat 2 tablespoons olive oil in a large ovenproof skillet over medium-high heat.

3. Add the mushrooms and sauté for 10 minutes, until golden brown and lightly caramelized.

4. Add the garlic and thyme and sauté 2 minutes more.

5. Remove the mushrooms to a plate, cover with foil, and set aside.

6. Return the skillet to the heat and add the remaining olive oil.

7. Season the chicken thighs with salt and pepper.

8. Pan sear the chicken until lightly browned on both sides, about 10 minutes.

9. Place the skillet in the oven and roast until the chicken is cooked through, 20 to 25 minutes.

10. Serve the chicken with a generous spoonful of sautéed mushrooms.

WEIGHT MANAGEMENT TIP: Use boneless skinless chicken breasts instead of thighs to cut calories, saturated fat, and total fat.

PER SERVING Calories: 468; Total fat: 34g; Saturated fat: 9g; Carbs: 3g; Fiber: 1g; Protein: 32g; Sodium: 132mg

MEDITERRANEAN TURKEY SKILLET

FERTILITY BOOST • INFLAMMATION FIGHTER • WEIGHT MANAGEMENT

5-INGREDIENT

SERVES 4
Prep time: 10 minutes
Cook time: 30 minutes

1 tablespoon olive oil

1 pound boneless skinless turkey breasts, cut into 1-inch chunks

2 red bell peppers, thinly sliced

1 tablespoon minced garlic

1 (28-ounce) can of sodium-free diced tomatoes

1 cup sodium-free chicken broth

Sea salt, for seasoning

Freshly ground black pepper, for seasoning

The scent of simmering garlic-infused tomato sauce will fill your entire house and call everyone early to dinner. Tender peppers and juicy chunks of turkey round out this tempting dish. If you want a more filling meal, serve it over quinoa or brown rice. Add a generous sprinkling of chopped parsley for a boost of vitamin K, C, and A.

1. Heat the olive oil in a large skillet over medium-high heat

2. Add the turkey chunks and sauté for about 15 minutes, until just cooked through and golden brown.

3. Remove the turkey to a plate with a slotted spoon.

4. Add the peppers and garlic to the skillet and sauté 4 minutes.

5. Stir in the tomatoes and chicken stock.

6. Bring the mixture to a boil and then reduce the heat to low and simmer 5 minutes.

7. Stir in the reserved turkey and simmer 5 minutes more.

8. Season with salt and pepper.

INFLAMMATION-FIGHTING TIP: Accent this dish with ½ teaspoon dried rosemary. The herb contains antioxidant compounds such as carnosic acid and carnosol. These compounds are thought to block the production of inflammation-causing cytokines in the body.

PER SERVING Calories: 228; Total fat: 4g; Saturated fat: 1g; Carbs: 10g; Fiber: 2g; Protein: 28g; Sodium: 102mg

BLACKENED TURKEY BREAST

FERTILITY BOOST · INFLAMMATION FIGHTER · WEIGHT MANAGEMENT

5-INGREDIENT

SERVES 4
Prep time: 10 minutes
Cook time: 30 minutes

1 teaspoon sweet paprika

½ teaspoon garlic powder

½ teaspoon onion powder

¼ teaspoon cayenne

⅛ teaspoon sea salt

⅛ teaspoon freshly ground black pepper

1 pound boneless, skinless turkey breast, cut into 1-inch thick cutlets

1 tablespoon olive oil

Blackened is a term that describes a spice mixture associated with Cajun food. It also refers to the charred look when meat, poultry, or fish is pan seared in a hot skillet. Paprika is a common spice in the mixture and is loaded with vitamin A, vitamin E, iron, and many antioxidants such as lutein and zeaxanthin.

1. Preheat the oven to 375°F.

2. In a small bowl, stir together the paprika, garlic powder, onion powder, cayenne, salt, and pepper.

3. Rub the turkey cutlets all over with the spice mixture.

4. Place a large ovenproof skillet over medium-high heat and add the olive oil.

5. Pan sear the turkey 5 minutes on both sides and then place the skillet in the oven.

6. Roast the turkey until golden brown and cooked through, about 20 minutes.

COOKING TIP: If you own a barbecue, try grilling the turkey instead of roasting it. Place the turkey on the grill for 20 minutes, turning once. Traditional "blackened" dishes are often prepared on the grill to create the desirable dark color.

PER SERVING Calories: 165; Total fat: 6g; Saturated fat: 1g; Carbs: 1g; Fiber: 0g; Protein: 26g; Sodium: 87mg

TUNISIAN TURKEY

FERTILITY BOOST · INFLAMMATION FIGHTER · WEIGHT MANAGEMENT

ONE-POT
BULK COOK

SERVES 4
Prep time: 10 minutes
Cook time: 30 minutes

1 tablespoon olive oil

20 ounces of boneless skinless turkey thighs, cut into large chunks

1 sweet onion, chopped

2 teaspoons minced garlic

2 teaspoons grated fresh ginger

2 ripe peaches, pitted and chopped

¼ cup sodium-free chicken stock

¼ cup golden raisins

1 teaspoon ground cinnamon

Pinch allspice

Turkey is not a North African ingredient, but the flavor of this bird goes beautifully with the warm spices and sweet dried fruit associated with Tunisian cuisine. Allspice is an important part of this fragrant dish; just a pinch of this pungent spice goes a long way. Allspice is a good source of many inflammation-fighting minerals and nutrients such as vitamin C, potassium, copper, zinc, calcium, manganese, and iron. It can also relieve premenstrual syndrome symptoms and reduce the risk of diabetes and high blood pressure.

1. Heat the olive oil in a large skillet over medium-high heat.

2. Add the turkey and brown the chunks on both sides, for about 6 minutes total. Set the chunks and the juices aside in a bowl.

3. Add the onion, garlic, and ginger to the skillet and sauté until lightly caramelized and softened, about 3 minutes.

4. Stir in the peaches, stock, and reserved turkey along with the juices in the bowl.

5. Reduce the heat to low and simmer for about 10 minutes, until the peaches are soft.

6. Stir in the raisins, cinnamon, and allspice.

7. Cook until the turkey is tender but also thoroughly cooked. Stir occasionally, about 10 minutes.

BULK COOKING TIP: Turkey thighs freeze beautifully because they don't dry out like the breasts of this bird. If doubling this recipe, double all the ingredients except the cinnamon: use just 1½ teaspoons in the larger recipe.

PER SERVING Calories: 239; Total fat: 7g; Saturated fat: 2g; Carbs: 19g; Fiber: 3g; Protein: 25g; Sodium: 84mg

EASY BRUSCHETTA TURKEY

INFLAMMATION FIGHTER • WEIGHT MANAGEMENT

5-INGREDIENT

SERVES 4
Prep time: 10 minutes
Cook time: 40 minutes

2 tablespoon olive
oil, divided

20-ounces boneless
skinless turkey breast, cut
into 4 equal portions

Sea salt, for seasoning

Freshly ground black
pepper, for seasoning

6 plum tomatoes, diced

¼ cup chopped red onion

3 tablespoons chopped
fresh basil

1 tablespoon
balsamic vinegar

The simplicity of the fresh ingredients in the bruschetta topping allows the flavor of the turkey to shine through. Unlike some of the other protein sources recommended in the PCOS diet, you don't need to purchase grass-fed birds to get the best quality. That's because turkeys aren't grass fed. They're omnivores that eat bugs, seeds, feed, and even table scraps if offered to them. The best choice is an antibiotic, free-pasture-raised bird allowed to roam freely.

1. Preheat the oven to 400°F.

2. Heat 1 tablespoon olive oil in a medium oven-safe skillet over medium-high heat.

3. Season the turkey with salt and pepper.

4. Add the turkey to the pan and brown the turkey on both sides, about 8 minutes total.

5. Cover the skillet and bake the turkey for 25 to 30 minutes, until it's cooked through.

6. While the turkey is baking, stir together the tomatoes, onion, basil, balsamic vinegar, and 1 tablespoon olive oil in a small bowl.

7. Season the bruschetta with salt and pepper.

8. Serve the turkey topped with bruschetta.

INFLAMMATION BOOSTING TIP: There isn't a great deal of red onion in this colorful dish, so it is easy to substitute three shallots for the onion. Shallots contain higher quantities of vitamins, minerals, and antioxidants.

PER SERVING Calories: 237; Total fat: 8g; Saturated fat: 1g; Carbs: 10g; Fiber: 2g; Protein: 30g; Sodium: 138mg

TENDER TURKEY BURGERS

WEIGHT MANAGEMENT

BULK COOK

SERVES 4
Prep time: 15 minutes
Cook time: 30 minutes

2 teaspoons olive oil

½ sweet onion, chopped

½ red bell
pepper, chopped

1 celery stalk,
finely chopped

2 teaspoons minced garlic

1½ pounds ground turkey

Dash sea salt

Dash freshly ground
black pepper

Olive oil spray

4 sprouted grain buns

Boston lettuce leaves,
for garnish

Red onion, thinly sliced,
for garnish

Tomato, sliced, for garnish

Nothing is better on a balmy summer evening than enjoying juicy burgers on a balcony, patio, or deck with your family and friends. This recipe broils the patties, but they would be even more delicious on a barbecue, over medium heat, for about 8 minutes per side. Try sliced avocado and a spoon of salsa as a topping for a slightly more exotic meal.

1. Heat the olive oil in a medium skillet over medium-high heat.

2. Add the onion, red bell pepper, celery, and garlic and sauté until softened, about 4 minutes.

3. Transfer the cooked vegetables to a medium bowl and add the turkey, salt, and pepper.

4. Mix the ingredients together and divide the turkey mixture into four portions.

5. Shape the portions into four patties about ¾-inch thick.

6. Preheat the oven to 400°F.

7. Line a baking dish with parchment and place the turkey burgers on the dish in one layer.

CONTINUED

8. Lightly spray with olive oil.

9. Bake the burgers until they are golden and cooked through, about 25 minutes.

10. Serve the burgers on buns topped with lettuce, onion, and tomato.

BULK COOKING TIP: As with most burgers or ground meat creations, these patties freeze beautifully, either raw or cooked. Freeze the patties on a baking sheet before transferring them to a freezer bag. The raw patties can be cooked in the oven or on a grill right from the freezer.

PER SERVING Calories: 359; Total fat: 7g; Saturated fat: 1g; Carbs: 28g; Fiber: 5g; Protein: 47g; Sodium: 347mg

TURKEY CHIPOTLE CHILI

FERTILITY BOOST • INFLAMMATION FIGHTER • WEIGHT MANAGEMENT

ONE-POT
BULK COOK

SERVES 4
Prep time: 10 minutes
Cook time: 40 minutes

1 tablespoon olive oil

½ pound ground turkey

1 sweet onion, chopped

1 tablespoon
minced garlic

2 green bell
peppers, chopped

1 cup sodium-free red
kidney beans, drained

1 cup sodium-free
lentils, drained

1 (15-ounce) can
sodium-free diced
tomatoes

1 tablespoon chipotle
chili powder

¼ cup low-fat plain
Greek yogurt

2 tablespoons chopped
fresh cilantro

Chili is one of the most competitive dishes in culinary circles. Everyone has a perfect combination of protein, legumes (or no legumes), vegetables, spices, and toppings. Although turkey is probably not the first choice for many chili enthusiasts, this protein has a lovely mild flavor that soaks up the spices perfectly and combines well with any other additions to the dish. Turkey is a stellar source of protein and a crucial ingredient for fertility, about 30 grams in a 4-ounce portion.

1. Heat the olive oil in a large stockpot over medium-high heat.

2. Add the ground turkey and sauté until cooked through, about 7 minutes.

3. Stir in the onion and garlic and sauté for about 3 minutes, until softened.

4. Stir in the peppers, kidney beans, lentils, tomatoes, and chipotle chili powder.

5. Bring the chili to a boil, and then reduce the heat to low and simmer until the vegetables are tender and the flavors combine, about 30 minutes.

6. Serve topped with yogurt and cilantro.

BULK COOKING TIP: As with other heavily spiced recipes, do not double the chili seasoning along with the other ingredients. Start with 4 teaspoons chipotle chili powder. You can always strengthen the flavors when you reheat the recipe.

PER SERVING Calories: 280; Total fat: 6g; Saturated fat: 1g; Carbs: 35g; Fiber: 12g; Protein: 25g; Sodium: 277mg

CLASSIC TURKEY AND VEGETABLE SAUTÉ

FERTILITY BOOST · INFLAMMATION FIGHTER · WEIGHT MANAGEMENT

ONE-POT

SERVES 4
Prep time: 15 minutes
Cook time: 25 minutes

1 tablespoon olive oil

20-ounce boneless skinless turkey breast, cut into 1-inch chunks

1 sweet onion, cut into eighths

1 cup mushrooms, halved

2 teaspoons minced garlic

½ head broccoli, cut into florets

1 red bell pepper, diced

12 asparagus spears, cut into 2-inch pieces

½ cup sodium-free chicken stock

Sea salt, for seasoning

Freshly ground black pepper, for seasoning

This pretty assortment of vegetables and turkey chunks sauté together beautifully for a convenient one-pot meal that can be on the table in just over 30 minutes. Make sure you add the asparagus last so it does not get mushy and gray in color. Asparagus is a potent anti-inflammatory due to its high flavonoid and saponin content. Asparagus is also very high in zinc, copper, and vitamins A and C, which are excellent for fertility.

1. Heat the olive oil in a large skillet over medium-high heat.

2. Add the turkey and sauté for about 12 minutes, until it's cooked through and lightly browned.

3. Remove the turkey to a plate with a slotted spoon.

4. Add the onion, mushrooms, and garlic and sauté for about 6 minutes, until the vegetables are lightly caramelized.

5. Add the broccoli, red bell pepper, and asparagus and sauté for about 6 minutes, until the vegetables are tender crisp.

6. Add the chicken stock along with the reserved turkey and any accumulated juice from the plate.

7. Sauté for another 4 minutes and season with salt and pepper.

FERTILITY BOOST TIP: Double the asparagus in this dish if this tender vegetable is in season. The vegetable is an excellent source of folic acid. Healthy levels of folic acid can help decrease ovulation failure and boost fertility in women.

PER SERVING Calories: 225; Total fat: 5g; Saturated fat: 1g; Carbs: 14g; Fiber: 5g; Protein: 33g; Sodium: 138mg

TURKEY ZUCCHINI NOODLE BOWL

FERTILITY BOOST • INFLAMMATION FIGHTER • WEIGHT MANAGEMENT

30-MINUTE

SERVES 4
Prep time: 20 minutes
Cook time: 25 minutes

2 teaspoons sesame oil

1 pound boneless, skinless turkey breasts, cut into strips about 2-inches long

1 cup Tahini Peanut Sauce (page 188)

2 zucchini, cut into ribbons with a peeler or spiralized

3 carrots, julienned

1 red bell pepper, julienned

1 cup shredded kale

1 cup chopped broccoli

3 tablespoons chopped fresh cilantro

Bowls are a trendy way to serve an assortment of ingredients in a beautiful way. This bowl is colorful and stunning enough that you will want to take a picture of it before you dig in. Broccoli florets soak up the tasty sauce and add interesting texture to the dish. Broccoli contains sulforaphane, which is crucial for the production of an enzyme that protects cells from damage caused by insulin resistance.

1. Heat the sesame oil in a large skillet over medium-high heat.

2. Add the turkey and sauté for about 15 minutes, until it's browned and just cooked through.

3. Add the sauce to the skillet and simmer the turkey until the sauce thickens, about 8 minutes.

4. Remove the skillet from the heat and shred the turkey using 2 forks.

5. In a large bowl, toss together the turkey and sauce, zucchini, carrots, red bell pepper, kale, broccoli, and cilantro.

6. Serve warm or cold.

FERTILITY BOOST TIP: Add a cup of sliced white mushrooms to increase the vitamin D in this dish. Vitamin D can help prevent or reverse ovulation problems and eating mushrooms with a calcium-rich vegetable like kale can increase the absorption of the calcium.

PER SERVING Calories: 390; Total fat: 21g; Saturated fat: 4g; Carbs: 20g; Fiber: 5g; Protein: 32g; Sodium: 136mg

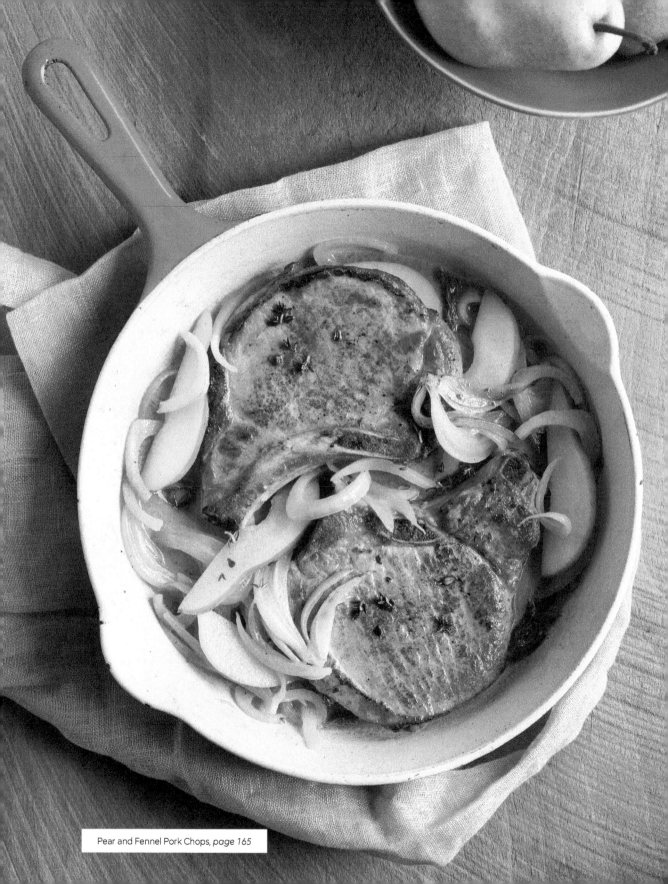

Pear and Fennel Pork Chops, *page 165*

BEEF AND PORK MAINS

FLANK STEAK
WITH ROMESCO SAUCE

INFLAMMATION FIGHTER • WEIGHT MANAGEMENT

30-MINUTE

SERVES 4
Prep time: 10 minutes
Cook time: 15 minutes

1 tablespoon olive oil, plus extra for greasing the rack

1 tablespoon minced garlic

1 cup roasted red pepper, chopped

½ cup almond flour

½ teaspoon smoked paprika

1 tablespoon apple cider vinegar

1 (1-pound) flank steak, trimmed

Sea salt, for seasoning

Freshly ground black pepper, for seasoning

Flank steak is not an expensive cut of meat like sirloin or tenderloin. It comes from the abdominal area of the cow and has long visible muscle fibers. This tougher cut of meat needs a little time in a marinade to tenderize. Flank steak can also be served with a slightly acidic sauce after you slice it very thinly across the grain. The apple cider vinegar in the Romesco sauce adds the right tartness to this dish. The roasted red pepper and smoky paprika add the appropriate balance. Leftovers can be wrapped in a sprouted grain tortilla the next day.

1. Preheat the oven to broil.

2. Place a rack on a baking sheet and lightly grease it with olive oil. Set aside.

3. Heat the olive oil in a small saucepan over medium-high heat.

4. Add the garlic and sauté for about 2 minutes, until softened.

5. Stir in the roasted red pepper, almond flour, paprika, and apple cider vinegar.

6. Heat until the sauce boils and then remove the saucepan from the heat.

7. Season the steak on both sides with salt and pepper.

8. Broil the steak to your liking; 5 minutes per side for medium-rare.

9. Remove the steak from the oven and let rest 10 minutes before slicing it thinly on a bias.

10. Serve with the sauce.

INGREDIENT TIP: Apple cider vinegar is a healthy addition to your PCOS diet because it can improve your body's sensitivity to insulin. This vinegar has a milder taste than distilled vinegar and a pleasing, slightly sweet flavor.

PER SERVING Calories: 340; Total fat: 19g; Saturated fat: 6g; Carbs: 4g; Fiber: 1g; Protein: 33g; Sodium: 256mg

CLASSIC KOFTE

INFLAMMATION FIGHTER • WEIGHT MANAGEMENT

30-MINUTE
BULK COOK

SERVES 4
Prep time: 15 minutes
Cook time: 15 minutes

1 teaspoon olive oil, for greasing the baking sheet

1 pound extra-lean ground beef

½ sweet onion, chopped

¼ cup almond flour

1 egg

3 tablespoons chopped fresh mint

2 teaspoons minced garlic

1 teaspoon ground cinnamon

4 (6-inch) sprouted grain pitas, split

2 tomatoes, chopped

¼ cup plain low-fat Greek yogurt

In North America, mint is often used only in desserts or sweeter dishes to accent chocolate or sugar. The herb is a very popular choice in savory recipes in other parts of the world such as the Middle East, Greece, and the Pacific Rim. The characteristically cool flavor of this gorgeous herb comes from a component called menthol, which can stimulate digestion and boost immunity. Mint is also very high in vitamins A, B_6, and C as well as iron, potassium, manganese, and magnesium.

1. Preheat the oven to broil.

2. Lightly oil a baking sheet with olive oil and set aside.

3. In a large bowl, combine the ground beef, onion, almond flour, egg, mint, garlic, and cinnamon.

4. Form the mixture into eight patties about ½-inch thick.

5. Place the patties on the baking sheet and broil until cooked through, about 6 minutes per side.

6. Stuff each pita bread half with one patty, tomato, and yogurt.

BULK COOKING TIP: To make extra, simply double the ingredients, including the spices, which are not used in large quantities in the original dish. The patties should be cooked before freezing. Thaw in refrigerator overnight and reheat at 400°F.

PER SERVING Calories: 300; Total fat: 9g; Saturated fat: 2g; Carbs: 23g; Fiber: 5g; Protein: 32g; Sodium: 270mg

MEDITERRANEAN-INSPIRED MEATBALLS

INFLAMMATION FIGHTER • WEIGHT MANAGEMENT

30-MINUTE
BULK COOK

SERVES 4
Prep time: 10 minutes
Cook time: 20 minutes

1 pound extra-lean
ground beef

1 egg

Juice and zest of 1 lemon

¼ cup chopped
fresh parsley

2 teaspoons minced garlic

2 teaspoons fresh
oregano, chopped

1 teaspoon prepared
horseradish

½ teaspoon ground cumin

¼ teaspoon sea salt

¼ teaspoon freshly ground
black pepper

The secret ingredient in the meatballs is a teaspoon of horseradish that brings a hint of heat. Horseradish is a natural antibiotic and contains more glucosinolates than broccoli. Horseradish can help reduce the risk of urinary tract infections, aid in digestion, and fight against infections and certain cancers. Eating horseradish can boost your immune system and contribute to good health.

1. Preheat the oven to 400°F.

2. Line a baking sheet with parchment and set aside.

3. In a large bowl, mix together the ground beef, egg, lemon juice, lemon zest, parsley, garlic, oregano, horseradish, cumin, salt, and pepper.

4. Roll the meat mixture into meatballs about 1-inch in diameter, and place them on the baking sheet.

5. Bake for about 20 minutes, until cooked through and golden.

BULK COOKING TIP: Cooked meatballs can be frozen on baking sheets and placed in plastic freezer bags. Use the extras for pastas, main meals, and soups. Thaw the meatballs in the refrigerator overnight and reheat them in sauce and soups so they stay juicy.

PER SERVING Calories: 173; Total fat: 6g; Saturated fat: 2g; Carbs: 2g; Fiber: 1g; Protein: 26g; Sodium: 200mg

BEEF-LENTIL RAGÙ

FERTILITY BOOST • WEIGHT MANAGEMENT

ONE-POT
BULK COOK

SERVES 4
Prep time: 15 minutes
Cook time: 1 hour,
25 minutes

1 tablespoon olive oil

6 ounces beef chuck
steak, trimmed and cut
into ½-inch chunks

1 sweet onion, chopped

2 celery stalks, chopped

2 teaspoons minced garlic

1 cup sodium-free
beef stock

2 tablespoons sodium-free
tomato paste

2 cups cooked lentils

Sea salt, for seasoning

Freshly ground black
pepper, for seasoning

2 tablespoons chopped
fresh parsley

Beef often gets a bad reputation because large quantities of red meat are not considered healthy. In moderate amounts, beef is a good protein choice. Beef is high in fat-soluble vitamins, omega-3 fatty acids, and conjugated linoleic acid (CLA), which can contribute to proper hormone function and production. Beef is also a very good source of iron, a nutrient crucial for healthy fertility.

1. Heat the olive oil in a large saucepan over medium-high heat.

2. Add the beef chunks and brown each piece on all sides, about 2 minutes on each side for a total of about 7 minutes.

3. Transfer the beef to a plate with a slotted spoon.

4. Add the onion, celery, and garlic and sauté for about 4 minutes, until softened.

5. Stir in the beef stock, tomato paste, and beef, along with any accumulated juice from the plate, to the saucepan.

6. Bring to a boil, and then reduce the heat to low. Cover and simmer for about 1 hour, until the beef is tender.

7. Stir in the lentils and simmer for 15 minutes more.

8. Season with salt and pepper.

9. Serve topped with parsley.

BULK COOKING TIP: If you own a food processor, use it to chop your vegetables, especially if you plan to double or triple this recipe. Do not overcook the carrots, parsnip, and lentils because they can get very mushy when you reheat the stew.

PER SERVING Calories: 310; Total fat: 9g; Saturated fat: 2g; Carbs: 30g; Fiber: 12g; Protein: 27g; Sodium: 156mg

HARISSA BEEF

INFLAMMATION FIGHTER • WEIGHT MANAGEMENT

**30-MINUTE
ONE-PAN**

SERVES 4
Prep time: 5 minutes
Cook time: 10 minutes

Olive oil, for greasing
the rack

2 tablespoons harissa

1 pound flank
steak, trimmed

2 tablespoons chopped
fresh parsley

Cucumber sticks,
for serving

Harissa is red chili paste used extensively in North African and Middle Eastern cuisine. This condiment is made from smoked chiles, tomato, rose petals, garlic, olive oil, cumin, caraway, and mint. Most of the ingredients in harissa are anti-inflammatories and even a little of the paste can go a long way, both nutritionally and flavor-wise.

1. Preheat the oven to broil.

2. Place a rack on a baking sheet and lightly oil the rack with olive oil.

3. Spread the harissa on the steak.

4. Broil the steak until desired doneness, 5 minutes per side for medium-rare.

5. Remove the steak from the oven and let it rest 10 minutes before slicing it thinly on a bias.

6. Serve topped with parsley with the cucumber sticks on the side.

FERTILITY BOOST TIP: If you want to make a more traditional recipe, lamb is a marvelous choice instead of beef. Lamb is high in vitamin B_{12}, with over 50 percent of the daily recommended amount. A deficiency in this vitamin can interfere with ovulation or create absent ovulation. Adequate amounts of vitamin B_{12} can reduce the risk of miscarriage because it can increase the endometrium lining after the egg is fertilized.

PER SERVING Calories: 296; Total fat: 15g; Saturated fat: 6g; Carbs: 3g; Fiber: 0g; Protein: 35g; Sodium: 196mg

BEEF-STUFFED BELL PEPPERS

INFLAMMATION FIGHTER • WEIGHT MANAGEMENT

BULK COOK

SERVES 4
Prep time: 15 minutes
Cook time: 40 minutes

4 red bell peppers, tops
cut off, seeded with
membranes removed

1 tablespoon olive oil,
plus extra for greasing
the peppers

¾ pound extra-lean
ground beef

1 sweet onion, chopped

1 cup mushrooms,
chopped

2 teaspoons minced garlic

1 cup shredded spinach

1 cup cooked quinoa

Sea salt, for seasoning

Freshly ground black
pepper, for seasoning

This savory beef, quinoa, and vegetable filling tastes spectacular with the tender, sweet roasted red pepper containers. Red bell peppers, mushrooms, quinoa, and spinach can help lower blood sugar because they are high in vitamins A, C, and K. Add a touch of cinnamon if you want to increase insulin sensitivity in cells to make this meal even more of a healthy PCOS diet choice.

1. Preheat the oven to 350°F.

2. Rub peppers with olive oil and place them hollow side down in baking pan.

3. Bake the peppers for 10 minutes, until slightly softened, and remove them from the oven. Flip them hollow side up and set aside.

4. Heat the olive oil in a large skillet over medium-high heat.

5. Add the ground beef and sauté for about 10 minutes, until it is cooked through.

6. Stir in the onion, mushrooms, and garlic and sauté for about 6 minutes, until translucent.

7. Remove the skillet from the heat and stir in the spinach and quinoa.

8. Season the filling with salt and pepper.

9. Spoon the filling into the red peppers and return the baking dish to the oven.

10. Bake 15 minutes and serve.

BULK COOKING TIP: Stuffed peppers are a hearty but simple meal that can be made with any color bell pepper. Freeze the peppers after step 9 in the recipe, in either a disposable aluminum baking dish or individually in small plastic freezer bags. Thaw the peppers in the refrigerator before baking them for 20 to 25 minutes in a 350°F oven.

PER SERVING Calories: 239; Total fat: 8g; Saturated fat: 2g; Carbs: 18g; Fiber: 3g; Protein: 22g; Sodium: 121mg

CREAMY BEEF STROGANOFF

FERTILITY BOOST • WEIGHT MANAGEMENT

ONE-POT

SERVES 4
Prep time: 15 minutes
Cook time: 50 minutes

1 tablespoon olive oil

1 pound inside round beef, cut into thin strips

1 sweet onion, chopped

2 teaspoons minced garlic

2 cups mushrooms, sliced

2 cups sodium-free beef stock

2 tablespoons Dijon mustard

2 tablespoons cornstarch

½ cup low-fat plain Greek yogurt

Sea salt, for seasoning

Freshly ground black pepper, for seasoning

Beef and mustard is a culinary match made in heaven, especially Dijon, which has a sophisticated heat. Mustard is a Hindi symbol of fertility, so it should not be a surprise that it's rich in fertility-supporting nutrients such as selenium, omega-3 fatty acids, and manganese. Beef adds more to the combination with zinc, a mineral essential for balancing progesterone and estrogen as well as cell division. Zinc deficiencies are linked to early miscarriages.

1. Heat the olive oil in a large skillet over medium-high heat.

2. Add the beef and sauté for about 8 minutes, until browned.

3. Stir in the onion and garlic and sauté for 3 minutes.

4. Stir in the mushrooms and sauté for 5 minutes.

5. Add the beef stock and Dijon mustard and bring the liquid to a boil.

6. Reduce the heat to low and simmer for about 30 minutes, until the beef is very tender.

7. Stir the cornstarch into the yogurt and add the mixture to the stroganoff.

8. Stir for about 2 minutes, until the sauce thickens. Season with salt and pepper.

9. Serve over zucchini noodles or quinoa.

INFLAMMATION-FIGHTING TIP: White or button mushrooms are the traditional choice for stroganoff, but shiitake mushrooms can work well, too. Shiitake mushrooms can help inhibit oxidative stress because they contain a powerful anti-inflammatory called ergothioneine.

PER SERVING Calories: 240; Total fat: 8g; Saturated fat: 2g; Carbs: 13g; Fiber: 3g; Protein: 32g; Sodium: 247mg

BEEF AND VEGETABLE ROAST

INFLAMMATION FIGHTER • WEIGHT MANAGEMENT

ONE-PAN

SERVES 4
Prep time: 15 minutes
Cook time: 20 minutes

Olive oil, for greasing the baking sheet

1 head broccoli, cut into large florets

½ head cauliflower, cut into large florets

½ bulb fennel, coarsely chopped into 2-inch pieces

1 sweet onion, cut into eighths

2 teaspoons minced garlic

2 tablespoons olive oil

2 teaspoons fresh thyme, chopped

1 pound top sirloin steak, trimmed

Sea salt, for seasoning

Freshly ground black pepper, for seasoning

Make this meal once and you'll wonder why you've never created this one-tray preparation dish before. The steak cooks beautifully alongside the vegetables. The hint of herbs creates a bounty of fragrant flavors. Whenever possible, try to purchase grass-fed beef because it has double the amount of antioxidants such as lutein, beta-carotene, and carotenoids.

1. Preheat the oven to broil. Lightly oil a baking sheet and set aside.

2. In a large bowl, toss the broccoli, cauliflower, fennel, onion, garlic, olive oil, and thyme until well combined.

3. Spread the vegetables on the baking sheet, leaving room for the steak.

4. Season the steak with salt and pepper and place it on the baking sheet.

5. Broil the steak and vegetables until the steak is browned and the desired doneness, about 5 minutes per side for medium-rare. Stir the vegetables when you turn the steak.

6. Remove the steak from the baking sheet and let the meat rest for 10 minutes while you continue to roast the vegetables.

INFLAMMATION BOOST TIP: Toss six or seven peeled beets in with the other vegetables before roasting them. Beets are very rich in phytochemicals, such as carotenoids and flavonoids, as well as a powerful antioxidant and anti-inflammatory called betalain pigments. Betalain also boosts the metabolism and fights insulin resistance.

PER SERVING Calories: 254; Total fat: 12g; Saturated fat: 3g; Carbs: 14g; Fiber: 5g; Protein: 28g; Sodium: 180mg

ASIAN BEEF STRIPS

INFLAMMATION FIGHTER • WEIGHT MANAGEMENT

5-INGREDIENT

SERVES 4
Prep time: 10 minutes,
plus 30 minutes
marinating time
Cook time: 10 minutes

¼ cup coconut aminos

2 tablespoons rice
wine vinegar

2 tablespoons sesame oil

1 pound flank steak, cut
into ¼-inch wide strips

2 tablespoons
sesame seeds

These flavorful beef strips can be threaded onto skewers and grilled rather than broiled in the oven. If your skewers are made of wood, make sure you soak them in water for at least 30 minutes so they don't burn in the heat on the barbecue. In order to make slicing the steak easier, place the raw meat in the freezer until it is just firm.

1. In a medium bowl, stir together the coconut aminos, vinegar, and sesame oil.

2. Add the steak strips and stir to coat. Marinate the beef for 30 minutes at room temperature.

3. Preheat the oven to broil and place a rack on a baking sheet.

4. Arrange the beef strips on the rack and broil the steak, turning once, until medium doneness, about 10 minutes in total.

5. Serve topped with sesame seeds.

INFLAMMATION-FIGHTING TIP: Stir 2 tablespoons of raw honey into the marinade for a touch of sweetness and added proteolytic enzymes. The enzymes in honey can clear out cellular debris after breaking it down, which reduces inflammation in the body and boosts immunity.

PER SERVING Calories: 302; Total fat: 19g; Saturated fat: 1g; Carbs: 4g; Fiber: 1g; Protein: 25g; Sodium: 17mg

RESTAURANT STYLE PAN-SEARED STEAK

FERTILITY BOOST • WEIGHT MANAGEMENT

5-INGREDIENT
30-MINUTE
ONE-PAN

SERVES 4
Prep time: 10 minutes
Cook time: 10 minutes

2 (8-ounce) boneless
rib eye steak, about
1-inch thick

1 tablespoon olive oil

Sea salt, for seasoning

Freshly ground black
pepper, for seasoning

2 tablespoons chopped
fresh parsley

Many fine-dining restaurants do not have a grill in their kitchen. So to create juicy flavorful steaks, they sear the meat in cast iron pans on the range. This method allows all of the juices to stay in the pan and develop a wonderful caramelized crust on the meat. Beef is a great source of protein, which is crucial for fertility because amino acids are the building blocks for cells in the body and for the new cells during pregnancy.

1. Preheat the oven to 500°F.

2. Let the steak come to room temperature on a plate.

3. Place a large skillet, preferably cast iron, in the oven and let it heat up for 5 minutes.

4. While the skillet is heating up, oil the steaks with olive oil and season generously with salt and pepper.

5. Carefully remove the skillet from the oven and place it over high heat.

CONTINUED

6. Place the steaks in the skillet and pan sear for 1 minute. Turn the steaks over and pan sear 1 minute.

7. Place the skillet back in the oven and roast 4 minutes per side for medium doneness.

8. Remove the steaks from the skillet and let stand for 10 minutes before serving.

9. Serve thinly sliced on a bias topped with parsley.

INFLAMMATION-FIGHTING TIP: Use garlic-infused oil instead of regular oil, because garlic contains allicin, a powerful antioxidant compound. Allicin suppresses inflammation markers in the body and blocks enzymes that can increase an inflammation response.

PER SERVING Calories: 301; Total fat: 22g; Saturated fat: 9g; Carbs: 0g; Fiber: 0g; Protein: 20g; Sodium: 61mg

TOMATO BRAISED BEEF PATTIES

FERTILITY BOOST • INFLAMMATION FIGHTER • WEIGHT MANAGEMENT

5-INGREDIENT

SERVES 4
Prep time: 10 minutes
Cook time: 35 minutes

1 pound lean ground beef

Sea salt, for seasoning

Freshly ground black
pepper, for seasoning

1 tablespoon olive oil

1 sweet onion, chopped

1 (28-ounce) can
sodium-free diced
tomatoes

1 cup sodium-free
beef broth

3 tablespoons prepared
basil pesto

You will be reminded of meatballs in tomato sauce when you taste this easy, filling dish. Prepared basil pesto is a convenient condiment to have on hand to add flavor to your recipes. Basil is a good source of vitamin K, vitamin A, magnesium, and flavonoids. These nutrients protect against free radical damage and reduce inflammation.

1. Form the beef into four patties, about ½-inch thick, and season them lightly with salt and pepper.

2. Heat the olive oil in a large skillet over medium-high heat.

3. Add the burgers and cook until browned, about 5 minutes per side. Remove them to a plate and set aside.

4. Add the onion and sauté in the drippings for 3 minutes.

5. Stir in the diced tomatoes, beef broth, and pesto and bring the sauce to a boil.

6. Return the beef patties to the skillet, arranging them in one layer covered with sauce.

7. Simmer until the burgers are cooked through, about 20 minutes.

FERTILITY BOOST TIP: Stir 1 cup of green peas into the sauce, fresh or frozen, to increase the amount of zinc in the recipe. Zinc is crucial to produce hundreds of enzymes in the body, including those that keep estrogen and progesterone in balance.

PER SERVING Calories: 325; Total fat: 30g; Saturated fat: 7g; Carbs: 10g; Fiber: 2g; Protein: 25g; Sodium: 254mg

PORK WITH HOMEMADE APPLESAUCE

INFLAMMATION FIGHTER • WEIGHT MANAGEMENT

5-INGREDIENT
30-MINUTE
ONE-PAN

SERVES 4
Prep time: 5 minutes
Cook time: 25 minutes

1 pound pork tenderloin, cut on a bias into 12 pieces

Sea salt, for seasoning

Freshly ground black pepper, for seasoning

2 tablespoons olive oil, divided

2 apples, cored and chopped

¼ cup water

2 teaspoons raw honey

½ teaspoon ground cinnamon

Pinch ground cloves

Pork and apples are a classic combination that beautifully combines sweet and savory flavors. The apples in this recipe are not peeled, so you get the advantages of pectin, a soluble fiber, and quercetin, a powerful anti-inflammatory antioxidant. Make sure you scrub your apples well to remove any pesticides or other contaminants.

1. Lightly season the pork with salt and pepper.

2. Heat 1 tablespoon olive oil over medium-high heat.

3. Add the pork and panfry the pieces until just cooked through and golden brown, turning at least once, about 15 minutes in total.

4. Remove the pork to a plate and cover with foil to keep warm.

5. Add the remaining oil to the skillet and stir in the apples, water, honey, cinnamon, and cloves.

6. Sauté until the apples are tender and the water is evaporated, about 10 minutes.

7. Serve the pork topped with the apple mixture.

VARIATION TIP: Chops are also a nice cut to use in this recipe, especially boneless center cuts that are trimmed of fat. You will have to increase the cooking time by 5 to 10 minutes depending on how thick the meat is cut.

PER SERVING Calories: 250; Total fat: 11g; Saturated fat: 2g; Carbs: 19g; Fiber: 3g; Protein: 21g; Sodium: 286mg

SESAME-GINGER PORK CHOPS

INFLAMMATION FIGHTER • WEIGHT MANAGEMENT

5-INGREDIENT

SERVES 4
Prep time: 10 minutes,
plus 30 minutes
marinating time
Cook time: 20 minutes

2 tablespoons olive oil

1 teaspoon sesame oil

1 tablespoon grated
fresh ginger

2 teaspoons minced garlic

4 (4-ounce) boneless pork
chops, about 1-inch thick

2 tablespoons chopped
fresh cilantro

Pork, ginger, garlic, and sesame are a traditional combination found in many Asian-themed dishes. For extra flavor look for toasted sesame oil instead of plain sesame oil. Sesame oil is a wonderful source of copper, which is a natural anti-inflammatory.

1. In a medium bowl, stir together the olive oil, sesame oil, ginger, and garlic.

2. Add the chops, turning to coat, and marinate for 30 minutes.

3. Place a large skillet over medium-high heat and pan-fry the pork chops until golden brown and just cooked through, turning once, about 20 minutes in total.

4. Let the chops rest for 10 minutes.

5. Serve topped with cilantro.

FERTILITY BOOST TIP: Top the chops with a generous scattering of toasted sesame seeds to increase iron. Iron deficiency can cause irregular ovulation and decrease the quality of the eggs.

PER SERVING Calories: 197; Total fat: 11g; Saturated fat: 2g; Carbs: 1g; Fiber: 0g; Protein: 21g; Sodium: 287mg

TEX-MEX PORK TENDERLOIN

FERTILITY BOOST • WEIGHT MANAGEMENT

5-INGREDIENT

SERVES 4
Prep time: 10 minutes
Cook time: 30 minutes

1 cup Spicy Tex-Mex
Marinade (page 194)

2 (10-ounce) pork
tenderloins, trimmed
of visible fat

1 tablespoon olive oil

Pork is a healthy choice for protein and worldwide. It is consumed more than beef, lamb, or game meats. Pork is very high in B vitamins such as B_6 and B_{12}. Deficiencies in these vitamins can cause improper egg production and irregular menstruation. Pork is also a wonderful source of zinc, iron, protein, and thiamine.

1. Transfer the marinade to a large resealable bag and add the pork.

2. Seal the bag and marinate the meat in the refrigerator for 1 hour.

3. Preheat the oven to 400°F.

4. Heat the olive oil in a large oven-safe skillet over medium-high heat.

5. Take the pork out of the bag and discard the leftover marinade.

6. Place the pork in the pan and sear the pork for about 10 minutes, turning it until the meat is browned.

7. Place the skillet in the oven and roast until the pork is cooked through, about 20 minutes.

8. Let the cooked pork stand for 10 minutes before slicing.

FERTILITY BOOST TIP: Add a topping of chopped avocado to this spicy pork entrée to cool and enhance the flavors. One avocado adds 41 milligrams folic acid per serving as well as antioxidants, fatty acids, and potassium.

PER SERVING Calories: 227; Total fat: 7g; Saturated fat: 2g; Carbs: 8g; Fiber: 1g; Protein: 37g; Sodium: 125mg

SAVORY PORK VEGETABLE STEW

WEIGHT MANAGEMENT

ONE-POT
BULK COOK

SERVES 4
Prep time: 15 minutes
Cook time: 1 hour and
45 minutes

1 tablespoon olive oil

1 pound boneless pork
roast, cut into ½-inch
chunks

1 sweet onion, chopped

4 celery stalks, chopped

1 tablespoon
minced garlic

2 sweet potatoes, cut into
½-inch chunks

4 cups sodium-free
beef stock

6 ounces sodium-free
tomato paste

1 cup green beans, cut into
1-inch pieces

Sea salt, for seasoning

Freshly ground black
pepper, for seasoning

Pork stew is a nice change from the more popular beef version. It's perfect for chilly nights when you want a steaming bowl of hearty, stick-to-the-ribs ingredients. Carefully trim the pork roast to remove any visible fat or tendons. This will make sure the meat is fork tender after braising. This stew would be beautiful in a slow cooker as long as you do not stir in the green beans until the cooking time is complete.

1. Heat the olive oil in a large stockpot over medium-high heat.

2. And the pork and sauté for about 10 minutes, until the meat is browned all over. Using a slotted spoon, remove the pork to a plate.

3. Add the onion, celery, and garlic to the pot and sauté for about 4 minutes, until they soften.

4. Stir in the sweet potatoes and the reserved meat with any accumulated juice, beef stock, and tomato paste to the pot.

5. Bring the stock to a boil, and then reduce the heat to low. Simmer for about 1½ hours until the pork and vegetables are very tender.

6. Stir in the green beans and season the stew with salt and pepper.

BULK COOKING TIP: When doubling this recipe, omit the green beans from the portion you want to freeze; otherwise they will become mushy and turn an unappetizing grayish-green color when you reheat the stew.

PER SERVING Calories: 255; Total fat: 8g; Saturated fat: 2g; Carbs: 20g; Fiber: 5g; Protein: 25g; Sodium: 390mg

CINNAMON PORK SKILLET

INFLAMMATION FIGHTER • WEIGHT MANAGEMENT

ONE-POT

SERVES 4
Prep time: 10 minutes
Cook time: 1 hour

1 tablespoon olive oil

1 (1-pound) boneless pork roast, trimmed and cut into 1-inch cubes

1 sweet onion, chopped

1 tablespoon minced garlic

1 (15-ounce) can sodium-free diced tomatoes with the liquid

½ cup sodium-free beef stock

2 teaspoons ground cinnamon

½ teaspoon ground ginger

½ teaspoon sea salt

¼ teaspoon freshly ground black pepper

Cinnamon is often associated with sweet dishes, but the spice also works nicely with meats and poultry. Cinnamon can increase insulin sensitivity because it contains an active ingredient called hydroxychalcone. This warm spice also can stop postmeal sugar spikes because it can affect the speed at which food leaves the stomach. Look for Ceylon cinnamon because Cassia cinnamon is high in coumarin, which is known to contribute to liver damage.

1. Heat the olive oil in a large skillet over medium-high heat.

2. Add the pork cubes and sauté for about 10 minutes, until they are browned.

3. Add the onion and garlic and sauté 3 minutes.

4. Stir in the tomatoes, beef stock, cinnamon, ginger, salt, and pepper.

5. Bring the stew to a boil, then reduce the heat to low. Cover and simmer for about 45 minutes, until the pork is very tender.

INFLAMMATION-FIGHTING TIP: Although cinnamon is the dominant spice in this recipe, the ginger adds complexity and heat to the dish. Ginger is an antioxidant and anti-inflammatory. The spice contains a compound called gingerols, which can block the enzymes that can create inflammation in the body.

PER SERVING Calories: 186; Total fat: 6g; Saturated fat: 2g; Carbs: 8g; Fiber: 3g; Protein: 25g; Sodium: 301mg

PAN-SEARED PORK WITH BLACK OLIVE TAPENADE

FERTILITY BOOST • INFLAMMATION FIGHTER • WEIGHT MANAGEMENT

30-MINUTE

SERVES 4
Prep time: 5 minutes
Cook time: 25 minutes

FOR THE TAPENADE

½ cup pitted
Kalamata olives

¼ cup chopped
fresh parsley

2 garlic cloves

Juice and zest of 1 lime

1 tablespoon olive oil

FOR THE PORK CHOPS

4 (5-ounce) pork chops

Sea salt, for seasoning

Freshly ground black
pepper, for seasoning

2 teaspoons olive oil

Tapenade is a thick purée created using olives, garlic, herbs, and olive oil. Sometimes anchovies are blended in, but not in this version. Make the tapenade ahead of time and let it sit for at least 2 hours; the flavors will mellow beautifully. Kalamata olives are very high in polyphenols, which can lower the blood levels of C-reactive protein, which in turn lowers inflammation in the body.

FOR THE TAPENADE

1. Put the olives, parsley, garlic, lime juice, lime zest, and olive oil in a blender and pulse until the mixture is well combined but chunky.

2. Set aside.

FOR THE PORK CHOPS

1. Preheat the oven to 450°F.

2. Season the pork with salt and pepper.

3. Place a large oven-safe skillet over medium-high heat and add the olive oil.

4. Add the pork chops. Pan sear on both sides until browned, about 10 minutes in total, and place them in a baking dish.

CONTINUED

5. Bake the chops for about 15 minutes, until they are cooked through but still juicy.

6. Let the pork rest for 10 minutes and serve topped with the black olive tapenade.

FERTILITY TIP: Pork is often the second choice for many people after beef, but this protein source can be a great addition to your diet—in moderation. Pork is high in zinc, an important mineral for reproduction. Zinc can help promote correct cell division during conception and fetal development.

PER SERVING Calories: 317; Total fat: 22g; Saturated fat: 6g; Carbs: 3g; Fiber: 1g; Protein: 27g; Sodium: 643mg

PEAR AND FENNEL PORK CHOPS

INFLAMMATION FIGHTER • WEIGHT MANAGEMENT

ONE-POT

SERVES 4
Prep time: 10 minutes
Cook time: 35 minutes

1 tablespoon olive
oil, divided

4 (5-ounce) pork chops

Sea salt, for seasoning

Freshly ground black
pepper, for seasoning

2 pears, cored and
thinly sliced

½ fennel bulb, thinly sliced

½ sweet onion,
thinly sliced

½ cup sodium-free
chicken stock

2 teaspoons Dijon mustard

2 teaspoons fresh
thyme, chopped

The more traditional combination of apples and pork tastes delightful. The sweetness of the fruit complements the savory flavor of the meat. Pears work in a similar fashion and the licorice flavor of the fennel creates an interesting complexity. Pears are packed with soluble and insoluble fiber, and an assortment of flavonoids, such as flavan-3-ols, anthocyanins, and flavanols, which reduces the risk of insulin resistance.

1. Heat 2 teaspoons olive oil in a large skillet over medium-high heat.

2. Season the pork chops with salt and pepper.

3. Add the pork chops to the skillet and sear until just cooked through, about 10 minutes per side.

4. Remove the chops to a plate.

5. Add the remaining olive oil, and sauté the pears, fennel, and onion for about 10 minutes, until they are tender.

6. Stir in the stock and mustard and return the pork chops to the pan.

7. Cook until the liquid is reduced by half, about 5 minutes in total.

8. Serve topped with the thyme.

FERTILITY BOOST TIP: A teaspoon of ground cinnamon would add a warm and earthy flavor to this dish. Cinnamon supports healthy ovarian function and improves insulin resistance. As little as ½ teaspoon of this spice a day can significantly improve insulin resistance.

PER SERVING Calories: 342; Total fat: 17g; Saturated fat: 6g; Carbs: 21g; Fiber: 5g; Protein: 27g; Sodium: 532mg

GARLIC-HERB-MARINATED PORK

FERTILITY BOOST • INFLAMMATION FIGHTER • WEIGHT MANAGEMENT

5-INGREDIENT

SERVES 4
Prep time: 10 minutes
plus 1 hour marinating time
Cook time: 20 minutes

1 cup Mediterranean
Dressing (page 192)

4 (5-ounce) center-cut
loin pork chops

Sea salt, for seasoning

Freshly ground black
pepper, for seasoning

The garlic flavor in the dressing does not overpower the fresh herbs and sweetness of the balsamic vinegar. There is just enough of this allium to satisfy the senses and enhance the taste of the pork. Garlic is considered to be an anti-inflammatory superfood, but it also contains nutrients that boost fertility such as selenium. This mineral can assist in egg production and reduce the risk of miscarriage.

1. Place the dressing in a medium bowl and add the pork chops, turning to coat.

2. Place the bowl in the refrigerator to marinate for 1 hour.

3. Place a large skillet over medium-high heat.

4. Add the chops and pan sear for about 10 minutes each on both sides, until they are browned and cooked through.

5. Season with salt and pepper and serve.

INFLAMMATION-FIGHTING TIP: Garlic flavors this simple marinade recipe for the pork and adds a considerable amount of antioxidants. Garlic contains the compound allicin, which produces sulfenic acid when it's broken down in the body. Sulfenic acid rapidly neutralizes inflammation-causing free radicals in the body.

PER SERVING Calories: 209; Total fat: 9g; Saturated fat: 2g; Carbs: 1g; Fiber: 0g; Protein: 31g; Sodium: 129mg

GERMAN SAUERKRAUT AND PORK

INFLAMMATION FIGHTER • WEIGHT MANAGEMENT

ONE-POT

SERVES 4
Prep time: 10 minutes
Cook time: 1 hour and
40 minutes

1 (1-pound) boneless
pork shoulder roast

Sea salt, for seasoning

Freshly ground black
pepper, for seasoning

1 tablespoon olive oil

2 tablespoons
grainy mustard

1 (15-ounce)
jar sauerkraut, drained

½ cup sodium-free
chicken stock

Grainy mustard or pommery mustard has a distinctive texture because it is made with whole-grain mustard seed. Mustard is a member of the cruciferous vegetable family and has many of the nutrients associated with this superfood group. Mustard is a fantastic source of magnesium, selenium, and many phytonutrients that can reduce bodywide inflammation and provide pain relief.

1. Preheat the oven to 400°F.

2. Season the pork with salt and pepper.

3. Heat the olive oil in a large oven-safe skillet over medium-high heat.

4. Add the roast and brown on all sides, for about a total of 10 minutes.

5. Spread the mustard on the meat and arrange the sauerkraut around the meat.

6. Pour in the stock, cover, and roast in the oven until the meat is tender and cooked through, about 1½ hours.

7. Remove the cover in the last 20 minutes.

INFLAMMATION-FIGHTING TIP: Include fermented foods such as the sauerkraut in this recipe several times a week. These types of foods add beneficial bacteria to the gut. A healthy gut is crucial for reducing inflammation in the body. Sauerkraut can also assist the body with harmful toxin elimination.

PER SERVING Calories: 289; Total fat: 22g; Saturated fat: 7g; Carbs: 4g; Fiber: 2g; Protein: 21g; Sodium: 632mg

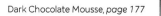
Dark Chocolate Mousse, *page 177*

SNACKS AND SWEET TREATS

SWEET POTATO DIP

INFLAMMATION FIGHTER • VEGETARIAN • WEIGHT MANAGEMENT

**30-MINUTE
ONE-POT**

MAKES 2½ CUPS
Prep time: 10 minutes

2 cups sweet potato,
cooked and puréed

½ cup plain low-fat
Greek yogurt

1 tablespoon raw honey

1 teaspoon pure
vanilla extract

¼ teaspoon ground
cinnamon

⅛ teaspoon
ground nutmeg

⅛ teaspoon ground ginger

Dash ground allspice

Fruit, for dipping

This dessert dip is the perfect snack when you're reading a book or watching a romantic comedy. Sweet potatoes are effective at reducing inflammation and keeping the blood sugar stable. This root vegetable is bursting with beta-carotene and vitamin A. It's also very high in vitamin C and manganese.

1. In a medium bowl, whisk together the sweet potato, yogurt, honey, vanilla, cinnamon, nutmeg, ginger, and allspice until well blended.

2. Serve with cut-up fruit.

3. Store the dip in a sealed container in the refrigerator for up to 1 week.

FERTILITY BOOST TIP: Winter squash is another inspired choice for this creamy dip. Squash adds almost 30 milligrams folic acid to each serving. Add 1 teaspoon of extra honey to the blend because squash is not as sweet as the potatoes.

PER SERVING (½ cup) Calories: 75; Total fat: 3g; Saturated fat: 2g; Carbs: 10g; Fiber: 1g; Protein: 2g; Sodium: 57mg

PUMPKIN AND SEED CRACKERS

INFLAMMATION FIGHTER • WEIGHT MANAGEMENT • VEGAN/VEGETARIAN

5-INGREDIENT
BULK COOK

MAKES 20 TO 24 CRACKERS
Prep time: 15 minutes
Cook time: 20 minutes

1¼ cups brown rice flour

½ cup flaxseed meal

¼ cup sesame seeds

2 tablespoons
poppy seeds

2 tablespoons flaxseed

½ teaspoon sea salt

¾ cup puréed pumpkin

These crackers deliver a double dose of flaxseed, so you get twice as much nutritional goodness. Flaxseed is loaded with magnesium, copper, manganese, phosphorus, thiamine, and fiber. It can aid in weight loss, lower bad cholesterol levels, and stabilize blood sugar.

1. Preheat the oven to 400°F.

2. Line a baking sheet with parchment paper and set aside.

3. In a large bowl, stir together the rice flour, flaxseed meal, sesame seeds, poppy seeds, flaxseed, and salt until well mixed.

4. Stir in the pumpkin and knead in the bowl until the ingredients are completely incorporated.

5. Transfer the dough to the parchment paper and use floured fingertips to spread the dough out flat. Place another piece of parchment paper on the dough and roll the dough out so it forms a rectangle about ⅛-inch thick.

6. Remove the top parchment paper and use a knife or pastry cutter to cut the dough into crackers about 2-inches square.

7. Bake the crackers until lightly golden, about 20 minutes.

8. Cool the crackers completely on the baking tray and then snap them apart.

9. Store the crackers in a sealed container in a dry cool place for up to 1 week.

BULK COOKING TIP: Once you taste these crispy beauties, you'll want them on hand for snacks at all times. You can freeze the crackers after they've completely cooled. If you double or triple the recipe, the crackers will keep for up to 1 month in the freezer. Just make sure they're stored in a freezer-safe bag.

PER SERVING (3 crackers) Calories: 172; Total fat: 6g; Saturated fat: 1g; Carbs: 22g; Fiber: 6g; Protein: 5g; Sodium: 6mg

SPICED MIXED NUTS

FERTILITY BOOST · INFLAMMATION FIGHTER · VEGETARIAN

BULK COOK

SERVES 10
Prep time: 10 minutes
Cook time: 35 minutes

1 cup almonds

1 cup pecans

1 cup cashews

½ cup hazelnuts

1 tablespoon
coconut aminos

2 teaspoons olive oil

2 teaspoons raw honey

1 teaspoon ground cumin

Pinch ground cayenne

Nuts are fabulous snack, but be sure not to overindulge as they're high in fat and calories. Nuts are rich in fiber and protein and healthy monounsaturated and polyunsaturated fats. They can lower blood sugar, lower bad cholesterol levels, reduce insulin resistance, and help you feel full longer. Use whatever combination of nuts you desire for this recipe.

1. Preheat the oven to 300°F.

2. Line a baking sheet with parchment, and spread the almonds, pecans, cashews, and hazelnuts on the sheet. Roast until crisp and golden, stirring frequently, about 20 minutes.

3. While the nuts are roasting, whisk together the coconut aminos, olive oil, honey, cumin, and cayenne in a small bowl. Set aside.

4. Reduce the heat to 250°F and remove the nuts from the oven.

5. Transfer the nuts to a large bowl and toss them with the coconut aminos mixture until well coated.

6. Return the nuts to the baking sheet and roast until the nuts are lightly caramelized, about 15 minutes.

7. Cool the nuts completely on the baking sheet and store in a sealed container in a cool, dry place for up to 5 days.

BULK COOKING TIP: Nuts are the perfect healthy snack when you need a quick energy boost or need to take the edge off your hunger pangs. If you double this recipe, use 1½ tablespoons coconut aminos, 1 tablespoon olive oil, 1 tablespoon honey, and 1½ teaspoons of ground cumin.

PER SERVING Calories: 232; Total fat: 19g; Saturated fat: 2g; Carbs: 9g; Fiber: 3g; Protein: 6g; Sodium: 103mg

FROZEN YOGURT BRITTLE WITH CHOCOLATE CHIPS

FERTILITY BOOST • WEIGHT MANAGEMENT • VEGETARIAN

5-INGREDIENT
NO COOK
BULK COOK

SERVES 8
Prep time: 15 minutes, plus freezing time

2 cups whole plain Greek yogurt

½ cup unsweetened shredded coconut

1 tablespoon raw honey

½ cup dark chocolate, finely chopped

It's difficult to describe the cool tart, slightly sweet flavor of this frozen treat; it's kind of a light chocolate-coconut cheesecake flavor. A full-fat yogurt is called for in this recipe. Fat isn't all bad, it plays an important role in the production of hormones, which are crucial for cell repair and for a healthy reproductive system. Eating healthy fats will also help you feel full longer and reduce your food cravings.

1. Line a baking sheet with parchment paper and set aside.

2. In a medium bowl, stir together the yogurt, coconut, and honey until well mixed.

3. Spread the yogurt mixture thinly on the parchment paper, about ¼ inch thick.

4. Sprinkle the dark chocolate evenly over the yogurt and place the baking tray in the freezer.

5. Freeze until completely frozen, about 3 hours.

6. Use a knife to break the brittle into pieces and store the brittle in the freezer in a sealed container for up to 1 month.

BULK COOKING TIP: If you double or triple the recipe, watch the quantity of honey so the yogurt isn't too sweet. Use 1½ tablespoons honey for a doubled recipe and 2 tablespoons for a tripled recipe.

PER SERVING Calories: 198; Total fat: 12g; Saturated fat: 10g; Carbs: 14g; Fiber: 2g; Protein: 5g; Sodium: 56mg

ENERGY COOKIES

FERTILITY BOOST • VEGETARIAN

30-MINUTE
BULK COOK

MAKES 16 COOKIES
Prep time: 10 minutes
Cook time: 10 minutes

¾ cup almond flour

½ cup rolled oats

½ cup sunflower seeds

½ cup dried cranberries
or blueberries

¼ cup shredded
unsweetened coconut

1 teaspoon ground
cinnamon

¼ teaspoon
baking powder

Pinch sea salt

½ cup natural peanut
butter

¼ cup raw honey

2 eggs

Cookies don't have to be empty-calorie snacks filled with sugar and unhealthy fat. They can also be loaded with ingredients that support a nutritious diet and boost your energy levels. These satisfying cookies contain nuts, seeds, dried fruit, and warm spices. The nuts can improve insulin sensitivity, reduce bad cholesterol, decrease free androgen amounts in the body, and bind testosterone to balance hormone levels.

1. Preheat the oven to 375°F.

2. Line a baking sheet with parchment paper and set aside.

3. In a large bowl, stir together the almond flour, oats, sunflower seeds, cranberries, coconut, cinnamon, baking powder, and salt.

4. In a medium bowl, whisk together the peanut butter, honey, and eggs.

5. Add the wet ingredients to the dry ingredients and stir to combine.

6. Drop the dough by tablespoons onto the baking sheets about 1-inch apart and bake until golden and firm, about 10 minutes.

7. Cool the cookies completely and store in a sealed container for up to 5 days.

BULK COOKING TIP: Freeze the cookies after cooling them completely in a sealed container for up to 1 month. The batter can also be frozen right on a baking sheet in tablespoon portions and then you can transfer them to a freezer bag. Remove the frozen batter and thaw on a baking sheet for an hour before baking them in a 350°F oven for 15 to 17 minutes.

PER SERVING Calories: 100; Total fat: 7g; Saturated fat: 2g; Carbs: 7g; Fiber: 2g; Protein: 5g; Sodium: 46mg

APPLE-CINNAMON BREAD

INFLAMMATION FIGHTER • VEGETARIAN

BULK COOK

SERVES 12
Prep time: 15 minutes
Cook time: 1 hour

Coconut oil, for greasing
the loaf pan

Gluten-free flour, for
dusting the loaf pan

½ cup granulated stevia

½ cup coconut oil

2 eggs

2 cups unsweetened
applesauce

2 cups almond flour

¼ cup rice flour

2 teaspoons
baking powder

1½ teaspoons ground
cinnamon

½ teaspoon sea salt

1 cup apples, peeled
and chopped

Coconut oil provides the crucial fat needed in this quick bread recipe. It helps create the structure of the bread and evenly distribute the sweetener throughout the batter. Coconut oil is the best choice, opposed to butter or other PCOS diet–friendly oils. It contains short- and medium-chain fatty acids, which are easily digested, taking the stress off of the pancreas, which increases the metabolic rate in the body, facilitating weight loss. Coconut oil is also linked to decreased inflammation and stable blood sugar levels.

1. Preheat the oven to 350°F.

2. Lightly grease a 9-by-5-inch loaf pan with coconut oil, dust it with flour, and set it aside.

3. In a large bowl, cream together the stevia and coconut oil with hand beaters until creamy, about 2 minutes, scraping down the sides of the bowl.

4. Add the eggs and beat to combine.

5. Beat in the applesauce, scraping down the sides of the bowl.

6. In a medium bowl, stir together the almond flour, rice flour, baking powder, cinnamon and salt until blended.

7. Add the dry ingredients to the wet ingredients and beat until just combined, scraping down the bowl with a spatula at least once.

CONTINUED

8. Stir in the apples and spoon the batter into the loaf pan and smooth the top.

9. Bake until a knife inserted into the center comes out clean, 50 minutes to 1 hour.

10. Cool the loaf for 30 minutes in the pan and then run a knife around the edges of the pan and pop the loaf out.

11. Cool completely on a wire rack and serve.

12. Store any extra wrapped in plastic wrap in the refrigerator for up to 5 days.

BULK COOKING TIP: Quick breads that freeze well are a favorite choice for many home bakers for easy entertaining. Make two loaves and freeze one so you can have some extra on hand. When doubling the recipe, increase all the ingredients by two, except the sweetener, salt, and cinnamon. Use ¾ cup sweetener, ¾ teaspoon salt, and 2 teaspoons ground cinnamon in the larger amount of batter.

PER SERVING Calories: 155; Total fat: 12g; Saturated fat: 8g; Carbs: 10g; Fiber: 2g; Protein: 2g; Sodium: 111mg

DARK CHOCOLATE MOUSSE

FERTILITY BOOST • INFLAMMATION FIGHTER • WEIGHT MANAGEMENT • VEGAN/VEGETARIAN

30-MINUTE
NO COOK

SERVES 4
Prep time: 10 minutes

1½ cups unsweetened almond milk

1 avocado

½ cup raw cashews

4 pitted dates

3 tablespoons cocoa powder

1 teaspoon pure vanilla extract

¼ teaspoon pure almond extract

As with many vegan or dairy-free desserts, puréed avocado provides the creaminess and thick smooth texture. Avocado is a PCOS superfood, with its powerful antioxidants such as omega-3 fatty acids, beta-carotene, lutein, and vitamin C. Avocado is also high in manganese, vitamin E, and selenium, which can help protect eggs from free radicals.

1. Place the almond milk, avocado, cashews, dates, cocoa powder, vanilla, and almond extract in a blender and pulse until the mixture is thick and creamy.

2. Transfer the mixture to four ramekins and chill in the refrigerator until you're ready to serve.

FERTILITY BOOST TIP: Cocoa is bursting with antioxidants, vitamins, and minerals such as iron and magnesium. Iron can help boost the low hemoglobin counts associated with PCOS heavy bleeding and magnesium improves insulin resistance.

PER SERVING Calories: 251; Total fat: 18g; Saturated fat: 4g; Carbs: 18g; Fiber: 6g; Protein: 5g; Sodium: 74mg

CHIA FRUIT PARFAIT

INFLAMMATION FIGHTER • WEIGHT MANAGEMENT • VEGETARIAN

NO COOK

SERVES 4

Prep time: 15 minutes, plus 4 hours thickening time

2 cups unsweetened almond milk

⅓ cup chia seeds

2 tablespoons raw honey

1 peach, chopped

½ cup strawberries, sliced

1 kiwi, chopped

¼ cup sliced almonds

¼ cup unsweetened shredded coconut

Parfaits seems like a dessert that should only be served in the summer on a shaded patio with a long-handled spoon in the glass. No matter what the season, this version will always be a welcome treat. The layered dessert features chopped fresh fruit such as a peach, strawberries, and tart kiwi. Kiwi can be either yellow or green with prominent black seeds and a fuzzy skin that should be peeled off. Kiwi is high in blood sugar–reducing fiber as well as vitamins A, C, E, and K.

1. Stir together the milk, chia seeds, and honey in a container and place the mixture, covered, in the refrigerator for at least 4 hours to thicken.

2. In a small bowl, toss together the peach, strawberries, and kiwi.

3. In four glasses, create parfaits by layering the ingredients in the following order: chia pudding, fruit, sliced almonds, chia pudding, fruit, and coconut.

INFLAMMATION-FIGHTING TIP: Use blueberries instead of the peach to add vitamin C and anthocyanins, an antioxidant. Anthocyanins can turn off inflammatory genes and vitamin C can help decrease free radicals in the body.

PER SERVING Calories: 288; Total fat: 20g; Saturated fat: 8g; Carbs: 26g; Fiber: 12g; Protein: 9g; Sodium: 96mg

GOLDEN SQUASH YOGURT CAKE

INFLAMMATION FIGHTER • WEIGHT MANAGEMENT • VEGETARIAN

5-INGREDIENT

SERVES 12
Prep time: 10 minutes
Cook time: 45 minutes

1½ cups butternut squash, cooked and puréed

2 cups plain low-fat Greek yogurt

½ cup almond flour

2 eggs

¼ cup raw honey

Pinch salt

This is more of a baked pudding than a cake. But the firm texture can be sliced, so the cake label is accurate. Butternut squash is moist and has a bright golden color, which indicates the presence of beta-carotene, a potent anti-inflammatory. Butternut squash is also a great source of omega-3 fatty acids, potassium, vitamin A, vitamin C, and folate. Add a generous heap of whipped coconut cream for a truly decadent treat.

1. Preheat the oven to 350°F. Line an 8-inch round cake pan with parchment and set aside.

2. In a large bowl, whisk together the squash, yogurt, almond flour, eggs, honey, and salt until smooth and thick.

3. Spoon the batter into the cake pan and bake until lightly golden brown, about 45 minutes.

4. Serve warm.

FERTILITY BOOST TIP: Ground flaxseed can be used instead of almond flour to increase the omega-3 fatty acids in the dish. Adequate levels of omega-3 fatty acids can decrease the risk of miscarriage and premature labor.

PER SERVING Calories: 80; Total fat: 2g; Saturated fat: 1g; Carbs: 11g; Fiber: 2g; Protein: 4g; Sodium: 52mg

SWEET POTATO PUDDING

INFLAMMATION FIGHTER • WEIGHT MANAGEMENT • VEGETARIAN

5-INGREDIENT

SERVES 8
Prep time: 10 minutes
Cook time: 45 minutes

½ cup melted coconut oil, plus extra for greasing the baking dish

5 cooked sweet potatoes, mashed

½ cup raw honey

4 eggs, beaten

½ cup freshly squeezed orange juice

Sweet potatoes and pecans are a traditional dessert pairing, especially in the South, so if you want a truly lovely dessert, top this pudding with a couple tablespoons of chopped pecans. More than 80 percent of the world pecan supply comes from 15 states in the United States and from trees that are over 100 years old. Pecans are extremely rich in folate, omega-3 fatty acids, fiber, and zinc. Pecans rank in the top 20 antioxidant-rich foods and contain the highest antioxidant content within the nut family.

1. Preheat oven to 350°F.

2. Lightly grease a 2-quart baking dish with coconut oil and set aside.

3. In a large bowl, stir together the mashed sweet potatoes, coconut oil, honey, eggs, and orange juice until smooth.

4. Pour into prepared baking dish and bake 40 minutes.

5. Serve warm.

FERTILITY BOOST TIP: The sweetener in this gorgeous dessert is honey, a traditional treatment for infertility in Ayurveda medicine, an ancient holistic treatment method. Honey can stimulate the ovaries and boost the level of antioxidants in the body.

PER SERVING Calories: 292; Total fat: 16g; Saturated fat: 12g; Carbs: 34g; Fiber: 6g; Protein: 4g; Sodium: 57mg

ALMOND-PEACH CUPCAKES

INFLAMMATION FIGHTER • VEGETARIAN

30-MINUTE

SERVES 12
Prep time: 10 minutes
Cook time: 20 minutes

1¾ cups almond flour

1 cup rice flour

½ cup stevia

2 teaspoons
baking powder

½ teaspoon baking soda

½ teaspoon
ground nutmeg

¼ teaspoon sea salt

1 cup coconut milk

⅓ cup melted coconut oil

2 eggs

2 teaspoons vanilla extract

2 cups chopped peaches

The tender crumb of these cupcakes is produced in part by the addition of creamy canned coconut milk. Shake the can well before you open it. The coconut cream will float to the top of the thinner milk if the can sits long enough. Coconut milk is a powerful anti-inflammatory made up of medium-chain triglycerides, so it can increase your energy levels and boost the immune system. This nutritious liquid also adds a delicate coconut flavor to the cake, which blends well with the almonds and peaches.

1. Preheat the oven to 350°F.

2. Line a 12-cup muffin tin with paper liners and set aside. In a large bowl, stir together the almond flour, rice flour, stevia, baking powder, baking soda, nutmeg, and salt until well blended.

3. In a medium bowl, whisk together coconut milk, coconut oil, eggs, and vanilla.

4. Add the wet ingredients to the dry ingredients and mix until combined.

5. Stir in the peaches and transfer the batter to the muffin pan dividing the batter evenly.

6. Bake until a toothpick inserted in the center comes out clean, about 15 to 20 minutes.

7. Serve after chilling on a wire rack.

VARIATION TIP: Exchange the peaches with nectarines, apples, or pears for a lovely change in texture and flavor. Look for fruit that is in season and peel the apples and pears.

PER SERVING Calories: 324; Total fat: 29g; Saturated fat: 24g; Carbs: 14g; Fiber: 2g; Protein: 3g; Sodium: 114mg

PEAR-COCONUT BUCKLE

INFLAMMATION FIGHTER • WEIGHT MANAGEMENT • VEGETARIAN

30-MINUTE

SERVES 8
Prep time: 10 minutes
Cook time: 20 minutes

FOR THE TOPPING
1 cup shredded
unsweetened coconut

½ cup almond flour

¼ cup coconut oil

1 tablespoon raw honey

½ teaspoon ground
cinnamon

Pinch salt

FOR THE FILLING
1½ pounds pears, peeled,
cored, and cut into
¼-inch slices

Pinch ground ginger

Coconut oil, to grease pan

Betty, buckle, crisp, and grunt—these are some of the different names used to describe fruit desserts baked with a crunchy or cakelike topping. The toppings can be made with breadcrumbs, nuts, oats, seeds, or a sponge cake, depending on the recipe and where it originated in the world. The base of this topping is nuts and shredded coconut, so you get all the anti-inflammatory benefits of these ingredients as well as from ground cinnamon and raw honey.

FOR THE TOPPING

1. In a medium bowl, stir together the coconut, almond flour, coconut oil, honey, cinnamon, and salt until the mixture resembles coarse crumbs.

2. Set aside.

FOR THE FILLING

1. Preheat the oven to 350°F.

2. Lightly grease a 9-by-9-inch baking dish with coconut oil.

3. Place the pears and ginger in the baking dish and toss.

4. Sprinkle the coconut topping on the pears and bake the pears until they are tender and the topping is crisp, about 20 minutes.

5. Serve warm.

FERTILITY BOOST TIP: Try stirring in ½ cup of cooked millet into the topping. This can help keep hormones in check by balancing insulin levels. Millet is an excellent source of fiber and iron, as well as vitamins E and B complex.

PER SERVING Calories: 162; Total fat: 11g; Saturated fat: 9g; Carbs: 16g; Fiber: 4g; Protein: 1g; Sodium: 23mg

CARROT SPICE CAKE

INFLAMMATION FIGHTER • WEIGHT MANAGEMENT • VEGETARIAN

BULK COOK

SERVES 16
Prep time: 15 minutes
Cook time: 1 hour

Coconut oil, for greasing
the cake pan

Almond flour, for dusting
the cake pan

1 cup melted coconut oil

¾ cup granulated stevia

3 eggs

2 teaspoons pure
vanilla extract

2 cups almond flour

1 cup oat flour

1 teaspoon baking soda

1 teaspoon ground
cinnamon

1 teaspoon baking powder

½ teaspoon sea salt

2 cups finely
shredded carrot

Carrot cake should be moist and spiced, and have bright shreds of carrot evenly distributed throughout each slice. Carrot is probably best known in nutrition circles as an excellent source of beta-carotene. It's also very high in other antioxidants. Carrots also contain anthocyanins and hydroxycinnamic acids to add to the anti-inflammatory effect of this bright vegetable.

1. Preheat the oven to 350°F.

2. Lightly grease a 9-inch round cake pan with coconut oil, dust it with flour, and set it aside.

3. In a large bowl, cream together the coconut oil and stevia with a hand mixer for about 2 minutes, until creamy, scraping down the sides of the bowl.

4. Add the eggs and vanilla and beat to combine, scraping down the sides of the bowl.

5. In a medium bowl, stir together the flours, baking soda, cinnamon, baking powder, and salt until blended.

6. Add the dry ingredients to the wet ingredients and beat until just combined, scraping down the bowl with a spatula at least once.

7. Stir in the carrots until just blended.

8. Spoon the batter into the cake pan and smooth the top.

9. Bake until a knife inserted into the center comes out clean, about 1 hour.

CONTINUED

10. Cool the cake for 20 minutes in the pan and then run a knife around the edges of the pan and pop the cake out.

11. Cool the cake completely on a wire rack and serve.

12. Store any extra wrapped in plastic wrap in the refrigerator for up to 5 days.

BULK COOKING TIP: This recipe also creates gorgeous muffins that are moist and pleasantly spiced. If you plan on doubling the recipe, it's best to mix up two individual batches of batter. Getting the correct amount of baking powder, baking soda, and spices is sometimes tricky. If those ingredients don't scale properly, it can lead to a flat and dense cake. If you make muffins, cook them for 25 to 30 minutes in a 350°F oven. Store them in sandwich bags in the freezer for up to 1 month.

PER SERVING Calories: 181; Total fat: 16g; Saturated fat: 12g; Carbs: 6g; Fiber: 1g; Protein: 3g; Sodium: 176mg

GOLDEN ANGEL FOOD CAKE

INFLAMMATION FIGHTER • WEIGHT MANAGEMENT • VEGETARIAN

5-INGREDIENT

SERVES 8
Prep time: 15 minutes
Cook time: 40 minutes

¾ cup potato starch

¼ cup cornstarch

1½ cups granular stevia

12 large egg whites,
at room temperature

½ teaspoon cream
of tartar

Angel food cake is a light, airy creation. It's made by beating air into egg whites and then gently folding them into the other ingredients. This process maintains the cake's volume. It can be labor intensive, but it's worth it in the end. The topping for this delight could be ripe, fresh raspberries and whipped coconut cream. Make sure you eat your raspberries within a day or two of purchasing them. Their high antioxidant content will degrade as they sit in the refrigerator.

1. Preheat the oven to 325°F.

2. Into a medium bowl, sift the potato starch, cornstarch, and sweetener. Set aside.

3. In a large bowl, beat the egg whites with the cream of tartar with a hand mixer for about 6 minutes, until stiff peaks form.

4. In four batches, gently fold the starch mixture into the egg whites.

5. Spoon the batter into an angel food pan and bake until the cake is golden brown and springy, about 40 minutes.

6. Remove the cake from the oven and cool completely in the pan.

7. Run a knife around the edge of the cake pan to remove the cake cleanly.

COOKING TIP: Do not beat the egg whites too much. Also, never grease the baking pan, because the angel food cake batter needs to cling to the sides as it rises.

PER SERVING Calories: 123; Total fat: 1g; Saturated fat: 0g; Carbs: 20g; Fiber: 2g; Protein: 7g; Sodium: 70mg

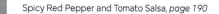
Spicy Red Pepper and Tomato Salsa, *page 190*

SAUCES, DRESSINGS, AND STAPLES

TAHINI PEANUT SAUCE

FERTILITY BOOST • INFLAMMATION FIGHTER • VEGETARIAN

30-MINUTE
NO COOK
ONE-POT

MAKES 1 CUP
Prep time: 10 minutes

½ cup creamy natural peanut butter

¼ cup tahini

1 tablespoon coconut aminos

1 tablespoon grated fresh ginger

Juice from 1 lime

1 teaspoon raw honey

1 teaspoon minced garlic

¼ teaspoon red pepper flakes

Tahini is a popular ingredient in Middle Eastern cuisine that can also be found in Balkan cuisine, Vietnamese cooking, and some Mediterranean dishes. It is made from toasted sesame seeds and has all the health benefits associated with the energy-packed seed. Tahini is a good source of copper, zinc, calcium, magnesium, and manganese. Minerals such as copper and zinc can help regulate ovulation.

1. In a medium bowl, stir together the peanut butter, tahini, coconut aminos, ginger, lime juice, honey, garlic, and red pepper flakes until well blended.

2. Transfer to a container and chill in the refrigerator.

3. Store the sauce in the refrigerator for up to 1 week.

INGREDIENT TIP: The coconut aminos in this sauce give it a distinct flavor very similar to soy or tamari sauces. You will find this ingredient in the organic food section of your grocery store.

PER SERVING (2 tablespoons) Calories: 262; Total fat: 20g; Saturated fat: 3g; Carbs: 9g; Fiber: 3g; Protein: 9g; Sodium: 135mg

PARSLEY-KALE PESTO SAUCE

INFLAMMATION FIGHTER • VEGAN/VEGETARIAN

5-INGREDIENT
30-MINUTE
ONE-POT
NO COOK
BULK COOK

MAKES 2 CUPS
Prep time: 10 minutes

1 cup fresh parsley

1 cup chopped kale

2 garlic cloves

¼ cup cashews

½ cup olive oil

Sea salt, for seasoning

Freshly ground black pepper, for seasoning

Pesto recipes are so popular it's almost impossible to read a cookbook without coming across another version. The sauce is popular for a good reason; the flavor is unbelievably addictive and simple to prepare. This recipe has a few changes from the traditional mixture. Instead of basil and pine nuts, it calls for parsley, kale, and cashews. The garlic in the recipe can help support a healthy gut, and reduce bad cholesterol and triglyceride levels.

1. Place the parsley, kale, garlic cloves, and cashews in a blender and pulse until the ingredients are finely chopped.

2. Drizzle the olive oil very slowly into the blender while it is running to form a thick creamy paste.

3. Season with salt and pepper.

4. Store the pesto in a sealed container in the refrigerator for up to 2 weeks.

BULK COOKING TIP: Pesto is incredibly versatile. Make extra and keep a jar handy for sauces, pasta, dressings, and main dish proteins. You can double this recipe with no changes, but if you triple it, use 5 garlic cloves instead of 6 unless you really like this ingredient.

PER SERVING (2 tablespoons) Calories: 71; Total fat: 7g; Saturated fat: 1g; Carbs: 2g; Fiber: 0g; Protein: 1g; Sodium: 20mg

SPICY RED PEPPER
AND TOMATO SALSA

INFLAMMATION FIGHTER • WEIGHT MANAGEMENT • VEGAN/VEGETARIAN

ONE-POT

MAKES 4 CUPS
Prep time: 10 minutes
Cook time: 45 minutes

2 pounds red bell
peppers, chopped

1 (28-ounce) can
sodium-free diced
tomatoes

1 sweet onion, chopped

1 jalapeño
pepper, chopped

2 tablespoons
minced garlic

2 tablespoons chopped
fresh cilantro

Juice of 2 limes

Sea salt, for seasoning

Freshly ground black
pepper, for seasoning

Many people with PCOS suffer from low iron. This can lead to anemia, which is a condition related to low red blood cells. Anemia can develop for many reasons, such as the body not producing enough red blood cells or because of heavy bleeding during menstruation. The tomatoes in this rich complex salsa are a wonderful source of vitamin C. These micronutrients help the body produce new red blood cells and support the synthesis of hemoglobin.

1. In a large saucepan over medium-high heat, stir together the bell peppers, tomatoes, onion, jalapeño, garlic, cilantro, and lime juice.

2. Bring the mixture to a boil and then reduce the heat to low. Simmer the salsa, stirring frequently, for about 45 minutes, until it is reduced by about half.

3. Transfer the salsa to a container and chill in the refrigerator.

4. Cover the salsa and store in the refrigerator for up to 2 weeks.

INFLAMMATION-FIGHTING TIP: Black pepper is often added as an afterthought to recipes and not considered to be a health benefit. The spice is also a powerful anti-inflammatory because of a chemical in it called piperine. The molecule reduces inflammation even in very small amounts. So, if you enjoy a little heat in your meals, give the pepper grinder a few extra turns.

PER SERVING (½ cup) Calories: 58; Total fat: 1g; Saturated fat: 0g; Carbs: 12g; Fiber: 3g; Protein: 2g; Sodium: 39mg

BLACKBERRY-POPPY SEED VINAIGRETTE

FERTILITY BOOST • INFLAMMATION FIGHTER • WEIGHT MANAGEMENT • VEGETARIAN

5-INGREDIENT
30-MINUTE
ONE-POT
NO COOK

MAKES 1½ CUPS
Prep time: 10 minutes

½ cup apple cider vinegar

½ cup fresh blackberries

1 tablespoon raw honey

1 tablespoon poppy seeds

¼ teaspoon chopped
fresh thyme

¾ cup olive oil

Sea salt, for seasoning

Blackberries are a succulent fruit: sweet, dark, and juicy. Like all other berries, blackberries are extremely high in antioxidants, specifically ellagic acid and anthocyanins, which is the source of its dark color. Blackberries are also a great source of blood sugar–stabilizing fiber and vitamins C and K. The berry can cut the risk of heart disease and diabetes as well as reduce the severity of PMS issues.

1. In a blender, combine the vinegar, blackberries, honey, poppy seeds, and thyme. Pulse until blended, about 30 seconds.

2. Pour in the olive oil and pulse until emulsified, about 15 seconds.

3. Season the vinaigrette with salt and store a sealed container in the refrigerator for up to 1 week.

4. Shake before using.

INFLAMMATION-FIGHTING TIP: The blackberries in this recipe give the dressing its exotic taste, but using fresh apricots would create another delicious iteration. Apricots contain quercetin, a phytochemical that can effectively fight inflammation in the body. Use the same amount of apricots as blackberries, about 3 or 4 in total.

PER SERVING (2 tablespoons) Calories: 121; Total fat: 13g; Saturated fat: 2g; Carbs: 2g; Fiber: 0g; Protein: 0g; Sodium: 20mg

MEDITERRANEAN DRESSING

INFLAMMATION FIGHTER • WEIGHT MANAGEMENT • VEGAN/VEGETARIAN

30-MINUTE
ONE-POT
NO COOK
BULK COOK

MAKES 1 CUP
Prep time: 10 minutes

¾ cup olive oil

¼ cup balsamic vinegar

1 tablespoon fresh oregano, chopped

1 tablespoon chopped fresh basil

1 teaspoon minced garlic

Pinch red pepper flakes

Sea salt, for seasoning

Freshly ground black pepper, for seasoning

This Greek-inspired dressing features a favorite herb from that region of the world: oregano. This unassuming herb contains one of the highest levels of antioxidants, ounce for ounce, of any food. Oregano contains a wide range of different antioxidants, so you get powerful protection from even a small amount. The herb is also nutrient-dense and a good source of fiber, vitamin K, manganese, and iron.

1. In a small bowl, whisk the olive oil and vinegar until emulsified, about 2 minutes.

2. Whisk in the oregano, basil, garlic, and red pepper flakes until well combined.

3. Season the dressing with salt and pepper and transfer to a container.

4. Store the dressing in a sealed container in the refrigerator for up to 2 weeks.

5. Shake before using.

BULK COOKING TIP: Double or triple the recipe. Then store the dressing in a clean empty wine bottle or decorative bottle in the refrigerator. Shake the dressing well and drizzle onto salads, fish, or side dishes.

PER SERVING (2 tablespoons) Calories: 166; Total fat: 18g; Saturated fat: 3g; Carbs: 1g; Fiber: 0g; Protein: 0g; Sodium: 32mg

HERB CITRUS SALT SUBSTITUTE

WEIGHT MANAGEMENT • VEGAN/VEGETARIAN

30-MINUTE
NO COOK
ONE-POT

MAKES ½ CUP
Prep time: 5 minutes

3 tablespoons dried basil

1 tablespoon dried thyme

1 tablespoon celery seed

1 tablespoon freshly
ground black pepper

1 teaspoon onion powder

½ teaspoon garlic powder

½ teaspoon lemon zest

½ teaspoon lime zest

½ teaspoon orange zest

Salt is not forbidden on a PCOS diet, but too much sodium can contribute to some of the chronic diseases that can be part of PCOS such as heart disease and stroke. Using a seasoning mix to replace salt in some recipes is a good culinary trick. This dressing has fragrant garlic and onion accents as well as a refreshing citrus undertone. It's perfect for seasoning vegetables, seafood, fish, poultry, and meats.

1. In a small bowl, stir together the basil, thyme, celery seed, black pepper, onion powder, garlic powder, and zests until well blended.

2. Store the seasoning in a sealed container for up to 2 weeks.

FERTILITY BOOST TIP: The herbs used in this mixture are only guidelines. Go ahead and experiment to see what combinations work best for your palate. Parsley is a good choice that marries well with the other herbs. The leafy herb is considered a traditional treatment for fertility issues. It's also rich in vitamin C, which has been used to help bring on menstruation.

PER SERVING (1 tablespoon) Calories: 8; Total fat: 1g; Saturated fat: 0g; Carbs: 1g; Fiber: 1g; Protein: 0g; Sodium: 2mg

SPICY TEX-MEX MARINADE

INFLAMMATION FIGHTER • WEIGHT MANAGEMENT • VEGAN/VEGETARIAN

30-MINUTE
ONE-POT
NO COOK

MAKES 1½ CUPS
Prep time: 10 minutes

½ cup olive oil

½ cup apple cider vinegar

¼ cup chopped
fresh cilantro

Juice and zest of 1 lime

2 teaspoons minced garlic

1 tablespoon cumin

1 tablespoon chili powder

2 teaspoons dried oregano

2 teaspoons freshly
ground black pepper

1 teaspoon ancho
chili powder

Marinades are a simple and effective method to get great flavor into proteins and also tenderize meat to improve texture. A mildly acidic blend is a favorite for marinades because the acid can break down the connective tissue found on tough cuts of meat. The trick is to marinade the protein for about 1 hour. Also make sure the acid isn't too strong or you end up with even tougher tissue. The apple cider vinegar in this marinade holds the perfect acidity level and comes with the bonus of improving postmeal insulin sensitivity.

1. In a medium bowl, whisk together the olive oil, vinegar, cilantro, lime zest, lime juice, garlic, cumin, chili powder, oregano, black pepper, and ancho chili powder until combined.

2. Store the marinade in a sealed container in the refrigerator for up to 1 week.

WEIGHT MANAGEMENT TIP: Apple cider vinegar can help manage weight, especially when ingested daily in small amounts, as little as 1 tablespoon per day. A study out of Japan looked at the acetic acid in apple cider vinegar, and their findings implied that the acid can turn on genes in the body that are responsible for triggering the enzymes that break down fat.

PER SERVING (2 tablespoons) Calories: 80; Total fat: 9g; Saturated fat: 1g; Carbs: 1g; Fiber: 1g; Protein: 0g; Sodium: 8mg

CHILI BARBECUE SAUCE

INFLAMMATION FIGHTER • WEIGHT MANAGEMENT • VEGAN/VEGETARIAN

ONE-POT

MAKES 2 CUPS
Prep time: 5 minutes
Cook time: 50 minutes

1 teaspoon olive oil

½ sweet onion,
finely chopped

1 tablespoon
minced garlic

½ cup water

½ cup sodium-free
tomato paste

¼ cup balsamic vinegar

1 chipotle pepper in
adobo sauce, chopped

1 tablespoon chili powder

2 teaspoons
Worcestershire sauce

¼ teaspoon ground
cinnamon

Sea salt, for seasoning

Freshly ground black
pepper, for seasoning

Homemade barbecue sauce is hard to beat. Most recipes are full of secret ingredients and techniques that only a few people know about. The idea is to produce an exclusive combination of sweet, savory, and smoky flavors. Barbecue sauce should be regularly prepared in almost every home kitchen because of its versatility. This recipe produces a sweet, tomato-based sauce with a smoky garlic finish that is perfect for meats, poultry, and vegetables.

1. Heat the olive oil in a medium saucepan on medium-high heat.

2. Add the onion and garlic and sauté for about 3 minutes, until softened.

3. Whisk in the water, tomato paste, vinegar, chipotle pepper, chili powder, Worcestershire, and cinnamon and bring the mixture to a boil.

4. Reduce the heat to low and simmer the sauce for about 45 minutes, stirring occasionally, until the flavors mellow.

5. Season the sauce with salt and pepper.

6. Transfer the sauce to a container and let it cool down before putting it in the refrigerator.

7. When the sauce is cool, cover, and store in the refrigerator for up to 1 week.

INFLAMMATION-FIGHTING TIP: Balsamic vinegar adds an incredible richness to this sauce; it's both bold and slightly fruity. This vinegar is also packed with an antioxidant called polyphenols that can decrease cell damage and boost the immune system. As little as 1 tablespoon per day of balsamic vinegar can positively affect insulin sensitivity.

PER SERVING (2 tablespoons) Calories: 12; Total fat: 0g; Saturated fat: 0g; Carbs: 2g; Fiber: 1g; Protein: 0g; Sodium: 51mg

STRAWBERRY JAM

INFLAMMATION FIGHTER • WEIGHT MANAGEMENT

5-INGREDIENT
BULK COOK

MAKES 2 CUPS
Prep time: 10 minutes,
plus 12 hours setting time
Cook time: 15 minutes

1 pound whole
strawberries, cleaned
and halved

1 tablespoon melted
coconut oil

1 (2-teaspoon) package
unflavored gelatin

2 teaspoons lemon zest

½ teaspoon ground
cinnamon

This jam recipe works well with any type of fruit. Peaches, apricots, cherries, plums, and other berries can be used individually or in a variety of mixtures. Strawberries are one of the most popular jam and jelly choices because they are sweet and create a glorious bright red spread. Strawberries are extremely high in antioxidants and can help reduce blood sugar levels.

1. Preheat the oven to 350°F.

2. Line a baking sheet with parchment paper and set aside.

3. In a large bowl, toss the strawberries and coconut oil.

4. Spread the berries on the baking sheet in one layer and bake until the berries are soft and lightly roasted, 15 to 20 minutes.

5. Transfer the berries back into the bowl and stir in the gelatin, lemon zest, and cinnamon.

6. Mash the berries with a potato masher until they are the desired consistency and the juices are thick.

7. Spoon the jam into a container and refrigerate for 8 to 12 hours so the jam sets.

8. Store the jam in a sealed container in the refrigerator for up to 2 weeks.

BULK COOKING TIP: Jam recipes can easily be doubled. But without preservatives, jams cannot be stored very long in the refrigerator. If you think you or your family can consume more than 2 cups of this spread in 2 weeks, then simply double the recipe and enjoy.

PER SERVING (2 tablespoons) Calories: 36; Total fat: 2g; Saturated fat: 2g; Carbs: 5g; Fiber: 1g; Protein: 1g; Sodium: 2mg

TART LIME CURD

FERTILITY BOOST · INFLAMMATION FIGHTER · WEIGHT MANAGEMENT · VEGETARIAN

5-INGREDIENT
30-MINUTE
ONE-POT

MAKES 1 CUP
Prep time: 5 minutes
Cook time: 10 minutes

½ cup freshly squeezed lime juice

¼ cup granulated stevia

Zest of 2 limes

4 large egg yolks

2 tablespoons coconut oil

It's no surprise that this rich tart topping and filling is very high in vitamin C. Limes, like all citrus fruits, are known for this potent antioxidant and can help reduce inflammation. Limes are a great source of folate, which can reduce the risk of certain birth defects and aid in healthy brain development in the womb.

1. Whisk together the lime juice, stevia, zest, and egg yolks together in a medium saucepan until well blended.

2. Place the saucepan over medium heat and continuously whisk until the mixture thickens, about 10 minutes.

3. Remove the saucepan from the heat and whisk in the coconut oil.

4. Transfer the curd to a container, cover tightly with plastic wrap, and cool the curd completely in the refrigerator.

FERTILITY BOOST TIP: Instead of lime, try creating an orange curd instead. Of all the citrus fruits, oranges are highest in folic acid. One medium orange contains about 29 milligrams folic acid. Use the same amount of juice and zest from one orange, but cut the sweetener to 1 tablespoon.

PER SERVING (2 tablespoons) Calories: 59; Total fat: 6g; Saturated fat: 4g; Carbs: 1g; Fiber: 0g; Protein: 1g; Sodium: 4mg

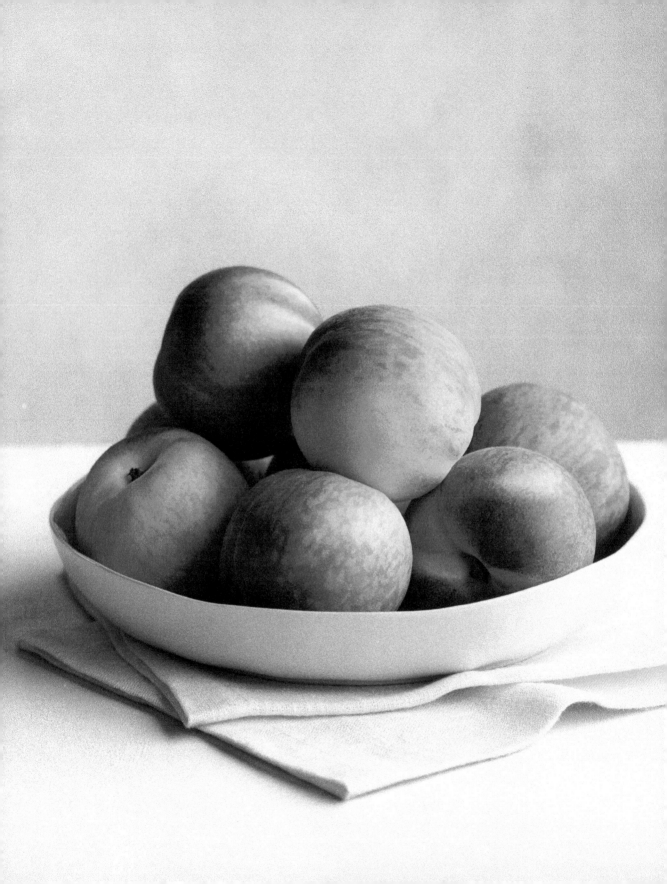

APPENDIX A: 2-WEEK MEAL PLAN WITH SHOPPING LISTS

Week 1 Meal Plan

Monday:

Breakfast: Hot Strawberry Breakfast Quinoa (page 29)

Lunch: Greek Chickpea Salad (page 46)

Dinner: Vegetable Baked Salmon (page 107)

Tuesday:

Breakfast: Kale-Pepper Egg Bake (page 26)

Lunch: Mixed Vegetable Lettuce Wraps (page 85)

Dinner: Mulligatawny Soup (page 38)

Wednesday:

Breakfast: PB&J Smoothie (page 21)

Lunch: Mulligatawny Soup (leftovers)

Dinner: Tender Turkey Burgers (page 137) (double recipe)

Thursday:

Breakfast: Apple-Cinnamon Bread (page 175)

Lunch: Tender Turkey Burgers (leftovers)

Dinner: Farmers Market Paella (page 89) (double recipe)

Friday:

Breakfast: Peach, Nut, and Sunflower Seed Muesli (page 30)

Lunch: Farmers Market Paella (leftovers)

Dinner: Beef and Vegetable Roast (page 153)

Saturday:

Breakfast: Chia Fruit Parfait (page 178)

Lunch: Red Lentil Pottage (page 40)

Dinner: Creamy Chicken Paprikash (page 126) (double recipe)

Sunday:

Breakfast: Mushroom Veggie Hash (page 31)

Lunch: Creamy Chicken Paprikash (leftovers)

Dinner: Quinoa Veggie Burgers (page 94) (double recipe)

Suggested Snacks:

- Zucchini-Wrapped Vegetable Rolls (page 62)
- Waldorf Smoothie (page 22)
- Ginger-Blueberry Smoothie (page 23)
- Crudité (carrots, celery, broccoli, and cherry tomatoes)
- Handful of assorted nuts

Week 1
Shopping List

Meat and Poultry

- Chicken thighs, boneless, skinless, 2 pounds
- Sirloin steak, 1 pound
- Turkey, ground, 3 pounds

Seafood

- Salmon fillets, 4 (6-ounce)

Dairy and Dairy Substitutes

- Almond milk, unsweetened, 4½ cups
- Eggs, 14
- Greek yogurt, low-fat, 3 cups

Produce and Herbs

- Apple, 2
- Bell pepper, red, 7
- Bell pepper, yellow, 1
- Bok choy, 5 small
- Boston lettuce, 2 heads
- Broccoli, 1 head
- Brussels sprouts, ½ pound
- Carrot, 3
- Cauliflower, 1 head
- Celery, 3 stalks
- Cherry tomatoes, 2 pints
- English cucumber, 1
- Garlic, minced, 9 tablespoons
- Ginger, fresh, 3-inch piece
- Green beans, 1 cup
- Kale, 1 head
- Kiwi, 1
- Lemon, 2
- Lime, 1
- Mushrooms, 2.6 ounces
- Onion, red, 2
- Onion, sweet, 13
- Peaches, 3
- Parsley, fresh, 1 bunch
- Spinach, 32 ounces
- Strawberries, 1 quart
- Thyme, fresh, 1 bunch
- Tomato, 3
- Wild mushrooms, 5.3 ounces
- Zucchini, green, 2
- Zucchini, yellow, 1

Regular Pantry Items

- Almond flour, 2 cups
- Almond slivers, ¼ cup
- Almonds, sliced, ¼ cup
- Applesauce, unsweetened, 2 cups
- Baking powder, 2 teaspoons
- Buns, sprouted grain, 8
- Cashews, chopped, 1 cup
- Chia seeds, ½ cup
- Chicken stock, sodium-free, 2 cups
- Chickpeas, sodium free, 2 (15-ounce) cans
- Cinnamon, ground, 2 teaspoons
- Cloves, ground, pinch
- Coconut, unsweetened shredded, ¼ cup
- Coconut oil, 9 tablespoons
- Coriander, ground, 1 teaspoon
- Cornstarch, 2 tablespoons
- Cumin, ground, 4 teaspoons
- Curry powder, 3 tablespoons
- Diced tomatoes, sodium-free, 2 (15-ounce) cans
- Flaxseed, 2 tablespoons
- Freshly ground black pepper
- Hazelnuts, chopped, 2 tablespoons
- Honey, raw, 5 teaspoons
- Nutmeg, ground, ½ teaspoon
- Oats, rolled, 1 cup
- Olive oil, 13 tablespoons
- Paprika, sweet, ¼ cup
- Peanut butter, natural, 2 tablespoons
- Peanuts, roasted and chopped, ¼ cup
- Quinoa, uncooked, 3½ cups
- Red lentils, dried, 3½ cups
- Red lentils, sodium-free, 3 (15-ounce) cans
- Rice flour, ¼ cup
- Sea salt
- Sesame seeds, 2 tablespoons
- Stevia, granulated, ½ cup
- Sunflower seeds, ¼ cup
- Tamari sauce, 4 teaspoons
- Vanilla extract, pure, 2 teaspoons
- Vegetable stock, sodium-free, 3 liters

Week 2 Meal Plan

Monday:

Breakfast: Kale-Pepper Egg Bake
(page 26)

Lunch: Quinoa Veggie Burgers
(leftovers)

Dinner: Savory Pork Vegetable Stew
(page 161) (double recipe)

Tuesday:

Breakfast: Apple-Cinnamon Bread
(page 175)

Lunch: Savory Pork Vegetable Stew
(leftovers)

Dinner: Classic Kofte (page 146)
(double recipe)

Wednesday:

Breakfast: PB&J Smoothie
(page 21)

Lunch: Classic Kofte (leftovers)

Dinner: Hearty Chicken Minestrone
(page 37)

Thursday:

Breakfast: Chia Fruit Parfait
(page 178)

Lunch: Hearty Chicken Minestrone
(leftovers)

Dinner: Navy Bean Shepherd's Pie
(page 87)

Friday:

Breakfast: Hot Strawberry Breakfast
Quinoa (page 29)

Lunch: Crunchy Asparagus-Cranberry
Salad (page 47)

Dinner: Seared Scallops with Warm
Coleslaw (page 105)

Saturday:

Breakfast: Mushroom Veggie Hash
(page 31)

Lunch: Wild Rice Peach Salad
(page 45)

Dinner: Tunisian Turkey (page 135)
(double recipe)

Sunday:

Breakfast: Peach, Nut, and Sunflower
Seed Muesli (page 30)

Lunch: Tunisian Turkey (leftovers)

Dinner: Spicy Crusted Haddock with
Citrus Basil Salsa (page 108) and
Spring Vegetable Mélange
(page 66)

Suggested Snacks:

- Green Citrus Smoothie (page 18)
- Lime-Fennel Smoothie (page 25)
- Energy Cookies (page 174)
- Peach or two plums
- A sprouted grain tortilla with
  almond butter

Week 2
Shopping List

Meat and Poultry

- Beef, ground, extra lean, 2 pounds
- Chicken, cooked, 2 cups chopped
- Boneless pork roast, 2 pounds

Seafood

- Haddock fillets, boneless, 4 (6-ounce)
- Sea scallops, 1 pound

Dairy and Dairy Substitutes

- Almond milk, unsweetened, 4½ cups
- Coconut milk, ¼ cup
- Eggs, 16
- Greek yogurt, low-fat, 1½ cups

Produce and Herbs

- Apples, 2
- Asparagus, 20 stalks
- Basil, fresh, 1 bunch
- Bell pepper, red, 2
- Bell pepper, yellow, 1
- Broccoli, 1 head
- Brussels sprouts, 1 pound
- Cabbage, green, 2 cups shredded
- Cabbage, red, ½ cup shredded
- Carrots, 3
- Cauliflower, 1 head
- Celery, 12 stalks
- Garlic, minced, ½ cup
- Green beans, 3 cups
- Jalapeño pepper, 1
- Kale, 1 bunch
- Kiwi, 1
- Mint, fresh, 1 bunch
- Onions, sweet, 7
- Orange, 1
- Oregano, fresh, 1 bunch
- Peaches, 5
- Pears, 2
- Red grapefruit, 1
- Scallion, 4
- Spinach, 32 ounces
- Strawberries, 1 quart
- Sweet potatoes, 6
- Tomatoes, 6
- White mushrooms, 5.2 ounces
- Wild mushrooms, 5.2 ounces
- Zucchini, yellow, 1

Regular Pantry Items

- Almond flour, 2½ cups
- Almond slivers, 6 tablespoons
- Apple cider vinegar, 5 tablespoons
- Applesauce, unsweetened, 2 cups
- Baking powder, 2 teaspoons
- Balsamic vinaigrette, 1 bottle
- Beef stock, sodium-free, 8 cups
- Caraway seed, ¼ teaspoon
- Chia seeds, ½ cup
- Chicken stock, sodium-free, 6 cups
- Chili powder, ½ teaspoon
- Cinnamon, ground, 1 tablespoon
- Cloves, ground, 1 pinch
- Coconut, unsweetened shredded, ¼ cup
- Coconut oil, ½ cup
- Cranberries, dried, ½ cup
- Diced tomatoes, sodium-free, 1 (28-ounce) can
- Flaxseed, 2 tablespoons
- Freshly ground black pepper
- Green peas, frozen, ½ cup
- Hazelnuts, chopped, 2 tablespoons
- Honey, raw, 5 tablespoons
- Navy beans, sodium-free, 1 (15-ounce) can
- Nutmeg, ground, ½ teaspoon
- Oats, rolled, 1 cup
- Olive oil, ¾ cup
- Peanut butter, natural, 2 tablespoons
- Pitas, sprouted grain, 8 (6-inch)
- Quinoa, dry, ½ cup
- Rice flour, ¼ cup
- Sea salt
- Sesame seeds, 2 tablespoons
- Stevia, granulated, ½ cup
- Sunflower seeds, ¾ cup
- Thyme, dried, 2 teaspoons
- Tomato paste, sodium-free, 12 ounces
- Vanilla extract, pure, 2 teaspoons
- Wild rice, uncooked, ½ cup

APPENDIX B: GLYCEMIC INDEX AND GLYCEMIC LOAD FOOD LISTS

The following is a list of the glycemic index and glycemic load rankings of many common carbohydrates. Foods are ranked between 0 and 100 based on how they affect one's blood glucose level. The best choices are foods that range between 55 to 69 on the glycemic index.

Remember that it is more important to pay attention to the glycemic load of a food—that is, the amount of carbohydrates it contains per serving. The best choices have low (less than 10) or moderate (between 10 and 20) glycemic loads.

FOOD	GLYCEMIC INDEX	SERVING SIZE grams, unless noted othewise	GLYCEMIC LOAD per serving
Bakery Products			
Bagel, white	72	70	25
Baguette, white	95	30	15
Barley bread	34	30	7
Corn tortilla	52	50	12
Croissant	67	57	17
Doughnut	76	47	17
Pita bread	68	30	10
Sourdough rye	48	30	6
Soya and linseed bread	36	30	3
Sponge cake	46	63	17
Wheat tortilla	30	50	8
White wheat flour bread	71	30	10
Whole-wheat bread	71	30	9

FOOD	GLYCEMIC INDEX	SERVING SIZE grams, unless noted othewise	GLYCEMIC LOAD per serving
Beverages			
Apple juice, unsweetened	44	250 mL	30
Coca-Cola	63	250 mL	16
Gatorade	78	250 mL	12
Lucozade	95	250 mL	40
Orange juice, unsweetened	50	250 mL	12
Tomato juice, canned	38	250 mL	4
Breakfast Cereals			
All-Bran	55	30	12
Cocoa Krispies	77	30	20
Cornflakes	93	30	23
Muesli, average	66	30	16
Oatmeal, average	55	50	13
Special K	69	30	14
Dairy			
Ice cream, regular	57	50	6
Milk, full-fat	41	250 mL	5
Milk, skim	32	250 mL	4
Reduced-fat yogurt with fruit	33	200	11
Fruits			
Apple	39	120	6
Banana, ripe	62	120	16

FOOD	GLYCEMIC INDEX	SERVING SIZE grams, unless noted othewise	GLYCEMIC LOAD per serving
Fruits, continued			
Cherries	22	120	3
Dates, dried	42	60	18
Grapefruit	25	120	3
Grapes	59	120	11
Mango	41	120	8
Orange	40	120	4
Peach	42	120	5
Pear	38	120	4
Pineapple	51	120	8
Raisins	64	60	28
Strawberries	40	120	1
Watermelon	72	120	4
Grains			
Brown Rice	50	150	16
Buckwheat	45	150	13
Bulgur	30	50	11
Corn on the cob	60	150	20
Couscous	65	150	9
Fettuccini, average	32	180	15
Gnocchi	68	180	33
Macaroni, average	47	180	23

FOOD	GLYCEMIC INDEX	SERVING SIZE grams, unless noted othewise	GLYCEMIC LOAD per serving
Grains, continued			
Quinoa	53	150	13
Spaghetti, white	46	180	22
Spaghetti, whole-wheat	42	180	26
Vermicelli noodles	35	180	16
White rice	89	150	43
Legumes			
Baked beans	40	150	6
Black beans	30	150	7
Butter beans	36	150	8
Chickpeas	10	150	3
Kidney beans	29	150	7
Lentils	29	150	5
Navy beans	31	150	9
Soy beans	50	150	1
Snack Foods			
Cashews, salted	27	50	3
Corn chips, plain, salted	42	50	11
Fruit Roll-Ups	99	30	24
Graham crackers	74	25	14
Honey	61	25	12
Hummus	6	30	0

FOOD	GLYCEMIC INDEX	SERVING SIZE grams, unless noted othewise	GLYCEMIC LOAD per serving
Snack foods, continued			
M&M's, peanut	33	30	6
Microwave popcorn, plain	55	20	6
Muesli bar	61	30	13
Nutella	33	20	4
Peanuts	7	50	0
Potato chips, average	51	50	12
Pretzels	83	30	16
Rice cakes	82	25	17
Rye crisps	64	25	11
Shortbread	64	25	10
Vanilla wafers	77	25	14
Walnuts	15	28	0
Vegetables			
Beets	64	80	4
Carrot	35	80	2
Green peas	51	80	4
Parsnip	52	80	4
Sweet potato, average	70	150	22
White potato, boiled	81	150	22
Yam	54	150	20

Sources: Harvard Health Publications (www.health.harvard.edu/healthy-eating/glycemic_index _and_glycemic_load_for_100_foods) and Mendosa.com (www.mendosa.com/gilists.htm).

APPENDIX C: **MEASUREMENTS AND CONVERSIONS**

VOLUME EQUIVALENTS (LIQUID)

US STANDARD	US STANDARD (OUNCES)	METRIC (APPROXIMATE)
2 tablespoons	1 fl. oz.	30 mL
¼ cup	2 fl. oz.	60 mL
½ cup	4 fl. oz.	120 mL
1 cup	8 fl. oz.	240 mL
1½ cups	12 fl. oz.	355 mL
2 cups or 1 pint	16 fl. oz.	475 mL
4 cups or 1 quart	32 fl. oz.	1 L
1 gallon	128 fl. oz.	4 L

VOLUME EQUIVALENTS (DRY)

US STANDARD	METRIC (APPROXIMATE)
⅛ teaspoon	0.5 mL
¼ teaspoon	1 mL
½ teaspoon	2 mL
¾ teaspoon	4 mL
1 teaspoon	5 mL
1 tablespoon	15 mL
¼ cup	59 mL
⅓ cup	79 mL
½ cup	118 mL
⅔ cup	156 mL
¾ cup	177 mL
1 cup	235 mL
2 cups or 1 pint	475 mL
3 cups	700 mL
4 cups or 1 quart	1 L

OVEN TEMPERATURES

FAHRENHEIT	CELSIUS (APPROXIMATE)
250°F	120°C
300°F	150°C
325°F	165°C
350°F	180°C
375°F	190°C
400°F	200°C
425°F	220°C
450°F	230°C

WEIGHT EQUIVALENTS

US STANDARD	METRIC (APPROXIMATE)
½ ounce	15 g
1 ounce	30 g
2 ounces	60 g
4 ounces	115 g
8 ounces	225 g
12 ounces	340 g
16 ounces or 1 pound	455 g

A nonprofit environmental watchdog organization called Environmental Working Group (EWG) looks at data supplied by the US Department of Agriculture (USDA) and the Food and Drug Administration (FDA) about pesticide residues. Each year it compiles a list of the best and worst pesticide loads found in commercial crops. You can use these lists to decide which fruits and vegetables to buy organic to minimize your exposure to pesticides and which produce is considered safe enough to buy conventionally. This does not mean they are pesticide-free, though, so wash these fruits and vegetables thoroughly.

These lists change every year, so make sure you look up the most recent one before you fill your shopping cart. You'll find the most recent lists, as well as a guide to pesticides in produce, at EWG.org/FoodNews.

DIRTY DOZEN

Apples	Nectarines	*In addition to the Dirty Dozen, the EWG added two types of produce contaminated with highly toxic organophosphate insecticides:*
Celery	Peaches	
Cherries	Spinach	
Cherry tomatoes	Strawberries	
Cucumbers	Sweet bell peppers	Kale/Collard greens
Grapes	Tomatoes	Hot peppers

CLEAN FIFTEEN

Asparagus	Eggplant	Onions
Avocados	Grapefruit	Papayas
Cabbage	Honeydew melon	Pineapples
Cantaloupe	Kiwis	Sweet corn
Cauliflower	Mangos	Sweet peas (frozen)

RESOURCES

The following list of additional resources provides more information about PCOS, insulin resistance, and how to prepare and cook meals.

Diabetes.co.uk is a global diabetes community that offers plenty of information about insulin resistance and prediabetes as well as dietary and lifestyle advice. www.diabetes.co.uk.

Jamie's Home Cooking Skills is the product of the chef Jamie Oliver. Offering step-by-step images and videos, it teaches inexperienced cooks everything from how to follow a recipe, prepare food hygienically, and safely handle a knife, and the difference between various cooking methods. www.jamieshomecookingskills.com /skills.php.

The **National Institute of Diabetes and Digestive and Kidney Diseases** website explains how insulin resistance and prediabetes develop, for those who would like to gain a better scientific understanding of their condition. www.niddk.nih.gov /health-information/health-topics/Diabetes/insulin-resistance-prediabetes.

The **Natural Fertility Info** website contains a comprehensive list of what supplements can help improve PCOS, and why. www.natural-fertility-info.com /pcos-fertility-diet.

PCOS Diet for the Newly Diagnosed is a book I wrote in 2017 that provides further details about the condition of PCOS and delves more into the nondietary ways of managing symptoms.

The **PCOS Awareness Association** is a nonprofit organization that aims to spread awareness about PCOS by increasing early diagnosis rates and overcoming the various individual symptoms of the condition. It links to a number of support groups worldwide. www.pcosaa.org.

The **PCOS Challenge** website is a national association for those with PCOS. It offers forums covering every topic from fitness, fertility, and PCOS-related depression, as well as blogs, videos, and recipes. www.pcoschallenge.org/pcos-support.

The **PCOS Diet Support** group is a community of women who are affected by PCOS. Within this Facebook group, the women share articles, general tips, and positive mantras to help one another overcome their PCOS. www.facebook.com /PCOSDietSupport.

The **PCOS Support Group** is an active community with almost 20,000 members who suffer from PCOS. https://pcos.supportgroups.com.

REFERENCES

Corbould, A. "Effects of Androgens on Insulin Action in Women: Is Androgen Excess a Component of Female Metabolic Syndrome?" *Diabetes Metabolism Research and Reviews* 24, no. 7 (October 2008): 520–532.

Hardy, O., Czech, M., and Corvera, S. "What Causes the Insulin Resistance Underlying Obesity?" *Current Opinion in Endocrinology, Diabetes and Obesity* 19, no. 2 (April 2012): 81–87.

Healthy Food Guide. "Food and PCOS: How Diet Can Help." Last modified February 2009. Accessed November 12, 2017. www.healthyfoodguide.com.au/articles/2009/february/food-and-pcos-how-diet-can-help.

Keller, U. "Dietary Proteins in Obesity and in Diabetes." *International Journal for Vitamin and Nutrition Research* 81, no. 2-3 (March 2011): 125–133.

King, R. "Factors Affecting Metabolism." *Drug Metabolism Handbook: Concepts and Applications* 10, no. 1002 (March 2010) doi:10.1002/9780470571224.pse101.

Kresser, C. "How Inflammation Makes You Fat and Diabetic (and Vice Versa)." Last modified September 15, 2010. Accessed February 5, 2017. www.chriskresser.com/how-inflammation-makes-you-fat-and-diabetic-and-vice-versa.

Lagana, A., Rossetti, P., Buscema, M., Vigneras, S., Condorelli, R., Gullo, G., Granese, R., and Triolo, O. "Metabolism and Ovarian Function in PCOS Women: A Therapeutic Approach with Inositols." *International Journal of Endocrinology* (August 2016): 1–9: doi:10.1155/2016/6306410.

Paddon-Jones, D., Westman, E., Mattes, R., Wolfe, R., Astrup, A., and Westerterp-Plantenga, M. "Protein, Weight Management, and Satiety." *The American Journal of Clinical Nutrition* 87, no. 5 (May 2008): 1558S–1561S.

Palsdottir, M. "Does Junk Food Slow Down Your Metabolism?" Healthline. March 21, 2017. Accessed November 16, 2017. www.healthline.com/nutrition/junk-food-and-metabolism.

PCOS Diet Support. "What Is the Best PCOS Diet?" Accessed November 12, 2017. www.pcosdietsupport.com/the-best-pcos-diet.

Traub, M. "Assessing and Treating Insulin Resistance in Women with Polycystic Ovarian Syndrome." *World Journal of Diabetes* 2, no. 3 (March 2011): 33–40.

RECIPE TYPE INDEX

5-Ingredient

Inflammation Fighter

Vegan

Weight Management

RECIPE TITLE INDEX

INDEX

ABOUT THE AUTHOR

Tara Spencer is a nutritionist and certified personal trainer who has worked with people from all walks of life. She encourages holistic, natural treatment methods for various kinds of illnesses. She is the author of *The Insulin Resistance Diet for PCOS*, *The Insulin Resistance Diet Plan and Cookbook*, and *The PCOS Diet for the Newly Diagnosed*.

CPSIA information can be obtained
at www.ICGtesting.com
Printed in the USA
LVHW051514190323
741874LV00001B/1